# Evidence-Based Medicine for PDAs
## A Guide for Practice

*Allan F. Platt, PA-C, MMSc*
Advanced Didactic Co-coordinator
Department of Family & Preventative Medicine
Emory University School of Medicine
Physician Assistant Program
Atlanta, Georgia

**JONES AND BARTLETT PUBLISHERS**
*Sudbury, Massachusetts*
BOSTON      TORONTO      LONDON      SINGAPORE

*World Headquarters*

Jones and Bartlett Publishers
40 Tall Pine Drive
Sudbury, MA 01776
978-443-5000
info@jbpub.com
www.jbpub.com

Jones and Bartlett Publishers
Canada
6339 Ormindale Way
Mississauga, Ontario L5V 1J2
Canada

Jones and Bartlett
Publishers International
Barb House, Barb Mews
London W6 7PA
United Kingdom

Jones and Bartlett's books and products are available through most bookstores and online booksellers. To contact Jones and Bartlett Publishers directly, call 800-832-0034, fax 978-443-8000, or visit our website www.jbpub.com.

Substantial discounts on bulk quantities of Jones and Bartlett's publications are available to corporations, professional associations, and other qualified organizations. For details and specific discount information, contact the special sales department at Jones and Bartlett via the above contact information or send an email to specialsales@jbpub.com.

The authors, editor, and publisher have made every effort to provide accurate information. However, they are not responsible for errors, omissions, or for any outcomes related to the use of the contents of this book and take no responsibility for the use of the products and procedures described. Treatments and side effects described in this book may not be applicable to all people; likewise, some people may require a dose or experience a side effect that is not described herein. Drugs and medical devices are discussed that may have limited availability controlled by the Food and Drug Administration (FDA) for use only in a research study or clinical trial. Research, clinical practice, and government regulations often change the accepted standard in this field. When consideration is being given to use of any drug in the clinical setting, the health care provider or reader is responsible for determining FDA status of the drug, reading the package insert, and reviewing prescribing information for the most up-to-date recommendations on dose, precautions, and contraindications, and determining the appropriate usage for the product. This is especially important in the case of drugs that are new or seldom used.

**Production Credits**

Executive Editor: David Cella
Acquisitions Editor: Kristine Johnson
Editorial Assistant: Maro Asadoorian
Production Director: Amy Rose
Production Editor: Renée Sekerak
Production Assistant: Julia Waugaman
Associate Marketing Manager: Lisa Gordon
Manufacturing and Inventory Supervisor: Amy Bacus
Composition: Auburn Associates, Inc.

Cover Design: Brian Moore
Cover Images: © Handy Widiyanto/
    ShutterStock, Inc.; © Johanna Goodyear/
    ShutterStock, Inc.
Chapter Opener Image: © Luis Francisco
    Cordero/ShutterStock, Inc.
Printing and Binding: Malloy Incorporated
Cover Printing: Malloy Incorporated

**Library of Congress Cataloging-in-Publication Data**

Platt, Allan F.
  Evidence-based medicine for PDAs : a guide for practice / by Allan Platt.
    p. ; cm.
  Includes bibliographical references and index.
  ISBN-13: 978-0-7637-5476-1 (pbk.)
  ISBN-10: 0-7637-5476-5 (pbk.)
  1. Evidence-based medicine—Data processing. 2. Pocket computers. I. Title.
  [DNLM: 1. Computers, Handheld. 2. Evidence-Based Medicine. 3. Medical Informatics Applications.
W 26.55.C7 P719e 2007]
  R723.7.P43 2008
  610.285—dc22
                            2007041989
6048

Printed in the United States of America
12  11  10  09  08      10  9  8  7  6  5  4  3  2  1

# Contents

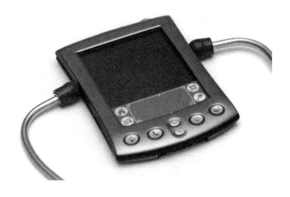

## Chapter 3 Differential Diagnosis and Physical Examination Tools for PDAs 29

## Chapter 4 Integrated EBM Programs 43

## Chapter 5 The Internet-EBM-PDA Web Sites 67

## Chapter 6 PDA Textbook Medical References 91

# Preface

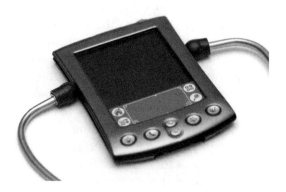

There is no single book available that gives medical practitioners or students the practical basics of PDA (personal digital assistant) computers and the evidence-based medical (EBM)
applications that are increasingly necessary to practice excellent patient care. Most clinicians have not had training using these new tools
and there are no textbooks for students covering these subjects for
medical programs. Medical informatics courses are only now beginning in the medical schools and physician assistant programs, but
there are no organized materials to help teach the courses.

This book is designed to be a resource for medical educators, students, and practicing clinicians who want to integrate EBM into their
daily practice in a practical way.

The main objective of this book is to introduce EBM as a strategy to
promote lifelong learning, continuing medical education, and high quality medical care based on the latest evidence. An additional benefit is
continuous study review for board examinations and potential CME credits. A glimpse into the future of PDAs will close the book. All the screen
shots in the book and video demonstrations will be on the Palm OS.

## Practicing EBM Every Day

Having a PDA on your belt or in your pocket allows you to conveniently
and rapidly look up questions as they arise in the clinic or hospital

setting. Getting into the habit of reviewing drug interactions and the latest treatments, and forming clinical questions, will keep you informed and learning every day. A medical practice is a fast paced environment, and clinicians do not have time to run to the office or library to read. Web access in the clinic or hospital setting can be spotty at best. Most clinicians do not have a list to review when they get home from a busy day, and medical reading is often pushed down on the priority list once the day is over. The ideal way to keep up during the workday is to do continuous information research in the spare minutes during and in between patient exams. To make this a reality, you need immediate access to a PDA, and you need programs that can be quickly accessed to answer your questions. The more you use these tools, the quicker you become, and the more this becomes a daily habit of lifelong learning.

When in the outpatient setting, read the chart before seeing your patient. Do a 2- to 3-minute lookup of any new or unfamiliar disease diagnoses to review the complications, prevention, and treatment options. The best references would be Epocrates Dx, Merck*Medicus*, Harrison's, or the *Merck Manual*. After taking the patient's history and while the patient is getting undressed for the physical exam, step out and do a 2- to 3-minute review of the chief complaint, differential diagnosis, and review the top possibilities. After the physical examination, step out of the room while the patient redresses and consult your PDA for the assessment, diagnostic tests, and treatment. Use the multidrug checker in either integrated product to make sure there are no hazardous interactions.

In the inpatient setting, while making rounds and doing chart reviews, look up the lab values and review the differential diagnosis. Look up unfamiliar diagnoses, and between patients, review the differential diagnosis for any new symptoms.

While in the emergency department, after obtaining the chief complaint of any unfamiliar problem, excuse yourself from the patient's side and do a quick review of the differential diagnosis using Epocrates Sx; read about the workup of the top diseases using Epocrates Dx or PEPID. After the history and physical exam, take a few minutes to review the studies needed and potential treatments using Epocrates Dx or PEPID. You may need a quick lookup using Epocrates Dx for an ICD-9 to add to the test requisitions. In formulating your treatment plan, use the multidrug checker in either integrated product to make sure there are no hazardous IV or oral drug interactions. In any free moment, review the ACLS and other emergency department protocols in either integrated product.

## The Remainder of the Book

This book is like a tool box with several hardware and software tools to bring the best evidence-based medical care to your patients. Chapter 1 gives an example of EBM using a PDA. Chapter 2 focuses on the tools and skills needed to get started. The hardware choices such as PDAs, phone-PDAs, wireless PDAs, Bluetooth, and beaming and peripheral equipment will be discussed. Software choices, Palm OS compared with Pocket PC, and bundled programs for word processing, spreadsheets, publishing, e-mail, pictures, Internet browsing, databases, and schedules also will be reviewed.

Chapter 3 discusses the software programs to aid in differential diagnosis. You cannot practice good EBM skills if you have the wrong diagnosis. A clinical case will be presented and the differential diagnosis tools will be demonstrated.

Chapter 4 compares two EBM-based integrated programs that combine differential diagnosis, drug, and lab, with interlinked medical reference text, and provide continuous updates: Epocrates Essentials and PEPID are the two leaders of integrated programs. All the aspects of each program will be demonstrated using clinical cases.

Because the Internet is critical for locating the latest clinical treatment information essential to practicing EBM, Chapter 5 covers this topic. Internet browsers, Web clipping programs, Internet search tools, and PDA-friendly medical Web sites for clinicians will be discussed.

Most of the major medical textbooks have a PDA version available, and Chapter 6 highlights this possibility. The most popular texts for EBM practice will be reviewed in a case-based approach.

Chapter 7 presents tools to assist with teaching, provides demonstrations to help teachers and students, and offers innovative ideas for integrating PDAs into the medical curricula.

Finally, Appendix A has a listing of general medical informatics Web sites and medical books about PDAs. Appendix B lists print resources for PDAs. A CD-ROM with interactive audio-visual video demonstrations using the hardware and software described in the previous chapters is also included.

# Acknowledgments

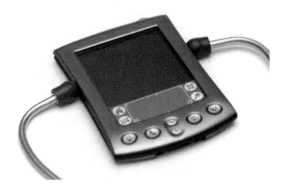

This book is a summation of a 20-year journey that satisfies my desire for all things medically geek. I wish to thank my wife Susan for putting up with my passion for computer gizmos. She is also one of my editors and physician reviewers who is a self-professed non-geek.

Thanks also to the Physician Assistant program at Emory University School of Medicine for allowing me the time to "git 'r done." A special thanks goes to the division director, Virginia Joslin, and faculty member Catherine Wilson for their reviews.

Thanks to Jones and Bartlett Publishers for making this book possible and to all the software developers creating all the great software that improves our clinical care.

The greatest thanks go to the maker of the best health insurance plan ever invented. No copays are involved and the premium is paid in full. The benefits are detailed in Psalm 103:1–5 (NIV):

Praise the LORD, O my soul;
all my inmost being, praise his holy name.
Praise the LORD, O my soul,

and forget not all his benefits—
who forgives all your sins
and heals all your diseases,
who redeems your life from the pit
and crowns you with love and compassion,
who satisfies your desires with good things
so that your youth is renewed like the eagle's.

*Allan Platt, PA-C, MMSc*

# CD-ROM
# Contents

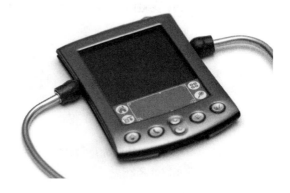

## Chapter 5 The Internet-EBM-PDA Web Sites



## Chapter 6 PDA Textbook Medical References



## Chapter 7 Teaching and Learning PDA-EBM Skills

# What Is Evidence-Based Medical Practice?

**1**

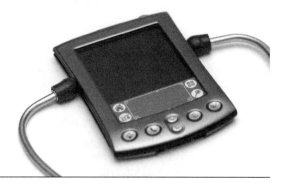

## Objectives

- Define and describe evidence-based medicine (EBM).
- Describe the importance of EBM in clinical practice.
- Describe how personal digital assistants can be EBM tools at the point of care.
- Use a case to demonstrate EBM principles.

## A Case to Solve

Mr. Smith, a 41-year-old male accountant, is in your office for a re-fill of his antihypertensive medication, hydrochlorothiazide 25 mg a day. He took his last pill this morning. He states he has been experiencing unilateral throbbing headaches that last about 1 to 2 hours. He has nausea and irritability prior to and during the headache. Bright lights aggravate the pain; taking ibuprofen and sitting in a dark quiet room help ease the pain. The headaches have occurred for years, but now they seem to happen weekly. The patient is having increased stress on the job. His blood pressure is elevated at 150/95 and the rest of his physical examination is normal. You only have a few minutes to gather your thoughts, write your notes, and present your plan to the patient. There is a computer with Internet access in the front office, but it is being used to check patient insurance status. There are a few textbooks in the office, but they were published a year ago.

- What is the differential diagnosis of the patient's headache?
- What is the best treatment for the patient's hypertension and headache?

## EBM in Motion

To approach the issues in this case, the clinician must know the differential diagnosis of headaches, the ramifications of being hypertensive and taking a diuretic and ibuprofen, and recommendations from the latest clinical trials regarding best treatment options for reducing the blood pressure and preventing the headaches. A personal digital assistant (PDA) in the clinician's pocket, with evidence-based medicine (EBM) software, could answer these questions in a few minutes, saving time, and provide a learning moment for the clinician.

This chapter will demonstrate how EBM references on a PDA could quickly provide the necessary information. Clinicians should know what types of PDA devices are available and be able to choose the best technology that is affordable, practical, and efficient. The next step is for the clinician to make the correct diagnosis. This involves his or her knowledge of differential diagnosis and clinical experience. New clinicians may have difficulty filtering a combination of many signs and symptoms. The experienced clinician knows which symptoms and signs may be causally related and the disease processes that produce them. Once a diagnosis—or a list of the most likely ones— is formulated, the clinician must focus on further diagnostic studies needed to finalize the diagnosis, treatment plans, and patient education. The experienced clinician may know all of the steps for common conditions seen on a routine basis, but a quick review or update of new therapy is needed to keep current. For the new clinician, guidance is needed to further the workup and treatment plan. Integrated EBM-PDA products are the best to use for quick lookups. If the patient has a condition not addressed by the integrated products, using the Internet with a wireless PDA is an excellent tool, allowing searches of large medical databases such as the National Library of Medicine or Clinical Guidelines. Some PDA programs allow Web clipping (copying pages of Web site information to the PDA for future reference) when wireless service is not available.

Paper textbooks of medicine usually take 2 to 3 years from the time of writing until they are edited and published. Most publishers are moving to e-textbooks that are available via the Internet, a personal computer (PC), and a PDA. The electronic book provides a subscription format with continuous updates so the information is searchable, linked to other resources, and never obsolete. These PDA books are great for obtaining more detailed information that is evidence based.

Teaching and learning about EBM using PDAs at the point of care is challenging to new and experienced clinicians alike. A case-based approach that simulates everyday practice is an excellent way to learn and teach about this new tool.

Sources through a PDA offer journal review, abstracts, and mobile continuing medical education credits so busy clinicians can keep up with the latest journal articles in their limited free time. This promotes lifelong learning and keeping current in the midst of a busy life. Clinicians can use PDAs and recommended programs to obtain continuing medical education credits and study for medical board examinations.

We now return to Mr. Smith in the examination room. After your physical examination, you step out of the examination room, pull your PDA from your coat pocket, and turn it on. An experienced clinician would have a good idea about the differential diagnosis, but a new clinician would appreciate the power of the symptom analyzer labeled Sx in the new Epocrates Essentials, a PDA medical reference software. A video demonstration of this case, labeled Video 1–1, is available on the CD-ROM.

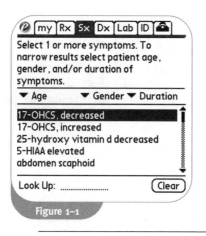

The first screen in the symptom analyzer allows the user to select the patient's age, gender, and duration of symptoms by tapping drop-down boxes.

Figure 1–1

my Rx Sx Dx Lab ID
Select 1 or more symptoms. To narrow results select patient age, gender, and/or duration of symptoms.
Age
Gender
Duration
< 2 mo
2 - 11 mo
1 - 11 yrs
12 - 17 yrs
18 - 40 yrs
41 - 65 yrs
> 65 yrs
Clear

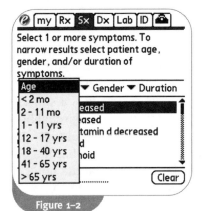

Figure 1–2

The age range for Mr. Smith is 41–65 years and he is a male, so tap each drop-down menu and select those choices.

---

my Rx Sx Dx Lab ID
Select 1 or more symptoms. To narrow results select patient age, gender, and/or duration of symptoms.
41 - 65 yrs
Male
Duration
17-OHCS, decreased
17-OHCS, increased
25-hydroxy vitamin d de
5-HIAA elevated
abdomen scaphoid
< 6 hrs
6 - 48 hrs
3 - 6 days
1 - 4 wks
> 4 wks
Look Up:
Clear

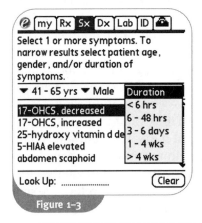

Figure 1–3

The duration is greater than 4 weeks.

---

my Rx Sx Dx Lab ID
Select 1 or more symptoms. To narrow results select patient age, gender, and/or duration of symptoms.
41 - 65 yrs
Male
> 4 wks
coital headache
headache
headache pounding
headache pulsating
headache throbbing
Look Up: heada
Clear

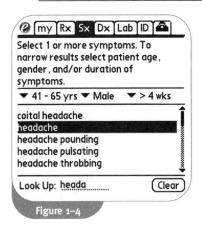

Figure 1–4

Then many symptoms and signs may be entered by keying the first few letters and tapping the correct word in the list that appears. For this example, choose “headache, throbbing.”

---

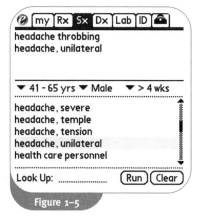

Figure 1-5

The next symptom to enter is the headache is unilateral. As you tap this from the choices, you will see it appear in the top list with the other symptoms and signs you have selected.

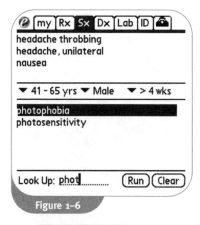

Figure 1-6

Enter nausea and photophobia and tap the Run box when you have finished entering all the signs and symptoms.

If you enter an item by mistake, just tap it in the upper list and it will be removed. The Clear button will remove all of your choices and allow you to start over.

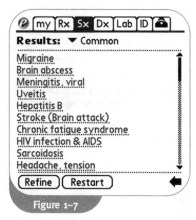

Figure 1-7

The symptom analyzer returns a list of the most common diagnoses based on the parameters and symptoms entered.

All of these disease choices are hyperlinked to full text descriptions in the Dx, or the 5-Minute Clinical Consult.

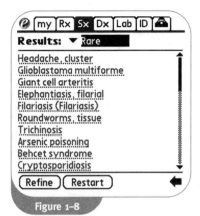

Figure 1–8

If you want to review a list of the rare causes, tap the common drop-down box and choose Rare. The list then appears.

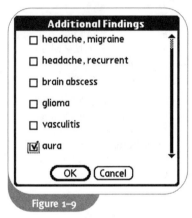

Figure 1–9

In the common list, you can tap the Refine box and a list of questions allows you to enter additional criteria. Your patient has recurrent headaches and says there is an aura of irritability preceding the pain.

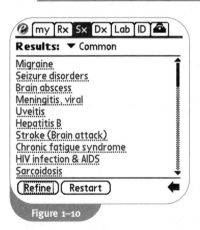

Figure 1–10

The differential list is further refined and Migraine has risen to the top choice. Each diagnosis is linked to an updated EBM reference, Dx, or the 5-Minute Clinical Consult. Tapping on Migraine links to a full review.

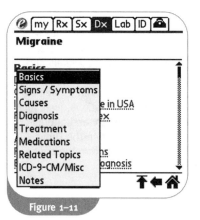

Figure 1-11

The 5-Minute Clinical Consult review has many sections to read. If you want to go directly to treatment options, tap that in the drop-down box.

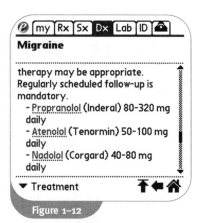

Figure 1-12

A list of medications appears that is specific to migraine prevention. Knowing that you need to add better blood pressure control, you tap on Atenolol, a selective beta-blocker.

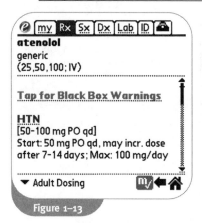

Figure 1-13

This is linked directly to the drug reference section that contains dosing information, warnings, side effects, and contraindications.

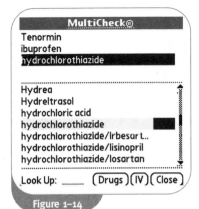

Figure 1-14

Tapping the M check in the bottom right corner of Figure 1-13 opens a drug multicheck program that allows the user to select potential as well as current medications, including complementary and alternative therapy. Tap the Drugs button to perform the multicheck.

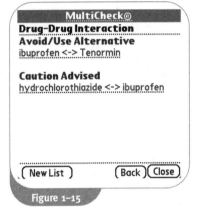

Figure 1-15

A list of cautions and contraindications appear for review. Tap on Drug–Drug Interaction for a text box with the caution.

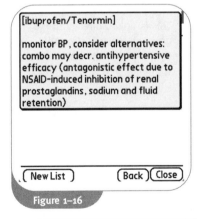

Figure 1-16

With this information, you will want an alternative to ibuprofen for the migraine pain.

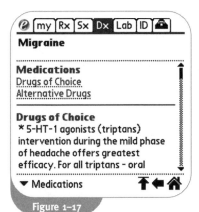

Figure 1-17

Go back to Dx and Migraine medications and you will see sumatriptan is the drug of choice. Tapping on this takes you back to RX.

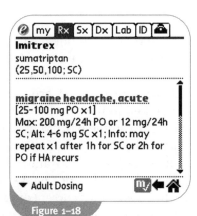

Figure 1-18

Entering all the medications now demonstrates no drug–drug interactions.

Tap the lower drop-down menu that has Adult Dosing and tap the Contraindications and Cautions option.

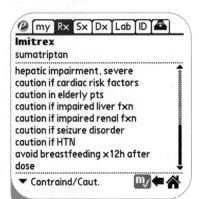

Figure 1-19

Sumatriptan must be used with caution in those with hypertension, but is not contraindicated.

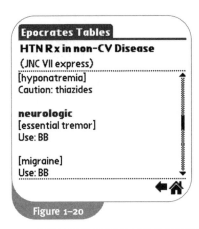

**Epocrates Tables**

**HTN R x in non-CV Disease**

(JNC VII express)

[hyponatremia]
Caution: thiazides

**neurologic**
[essential tremor]
Use: BB

[migraine]
Use: BB

Double check your idea with the JNC VII hypertension guidelines in the Tables section. You will see that for treating hypertension in the patient with migraines without cardiovascular disease, the best choice is a beta-blocker.

Figure 1–20

You can complete your write-up and plan with confidence that you have made the best choice of therapy with the least amount of potential side effects based on the latest evidence available. It is the author's opinion that this is one of the top integrated EBM-PDA programs, a combination of several modules interlinked to flow from one to another with a simple tap. This case was an example of EBM in motion using a PDA as a tool to access the latest treatment information.

If you did not have a PDA with these tools, you would wander down the clinic hallway to the bookshelf, hoping the reference books were current and look for a general medical textbook and a current drug reference. Most medical textbooks are organized by disease, so you would need a good differential diagnosis text to find the most likely disease. Most differential diagnosis texts are lists based on one major symptom. As a student, it is hard to know what symptom to look up. It should be the headache, but what about the nausea and photophobia? Is it related? Do you include the differential of nausea and the differential of photophobia and look where they all intersect? That would take a few extra minutes. Once you are sure about the diagnosis, you'll then look it up in the medical textbook. Here you should find the treatment plan, but know that a paper textbook is probably 2 to 3 years behind current research studies. Now that you have a medication in mind, it is time to open the drug reference. Looking up each medication and reading the indications and contraindications and side effects can take more precious minutes. To do a drug-to-drug interaction check would be nearly impossible if the patient were on three or more medications.

This quick case is an example of how a PDA with the right software can speed you along practicing excellent EBM in a very timely manner. The potential to reduce medication errors, practice daily lifelong learning, and provide the latest treatment is greatly enhanced.

## Evidence-Based Medicine

Evidence-based medicine is a continuous systematic review of the medical literature using the results of research studies to guide the patient workup and therapy. EBM was initially proposed by Dr. David Sackett and his colleagues at McMasters University in Ontario, Canada. Dr. Sackett defines EBM as ". . . the conscientious, explicit, and judicious use of current best evidence in making decisions about the care of individual patients" (Sackett, Richardson, Rosenberg, and Haynes, 1997).

Medical knowledge is increasing exponentially, and clinicians must practice lifelong learning skills to keep up with new treatments and diagnostic tests. Keeping up with medical journal articles and clinical trial results is unmanageable in the average clinician's daily practice, balancing medicine and personal time. A tool providing rapid references and answers to clinical questions at the point of care would allow clinicians to incorporate lifelong learning into their daily routine. Application of the latest medical evidence of best practice ensures excellence in patient care. This is the heart of EBM.

Classical EBM courses teach how to use epidemiology and biostatistical methods to appraise journal articles for the best evidence. There are several online courses such as the SUNY Downstate EBM Tutorial at http://library.downstate.edu/resources/ebm.html and the Center for Evidence Based Medicine at Oxford www.cebm.net/, Michigan State University at www.poems.msu.edu/InfoMastery/, and Duke University at www.hsl.unc.edu/services/tutorials/ebm/welcome.htm. These principles are valuable, but they are beyond the scope of this book. Our approach to EBM will be to review PDA products containing appraised medical literature. This provides the best evidence, making clinical recommendations for rapid reference at the bedside. With these products immediately accessible by PDA, clinicians should do

---

Sackett, DL, Richardson, WS, Rosenberg, W, Haynes, RB. *Evidence-Based Medicine: How to Practice and Teach EBM.* 1st ed. New York: Churchill-Livingstone; 1997, p 2.

lookups in their spare minutes while reviewing the chart before seeing the patient, as the patient undresses for the physical examination and after the examination while the patient dresses, and when formulating the notes and plan. This can only occur if the PDA resources are attached, as with a cell phone or in a coat pocket. The larger the device, the more inconvenient it is to carry, and the harder it is to do a quick lookup, the less likely it will be used and those EBM moments will be missed. Convenience encourages frequent lookups, updated practice habits, and continuous learning.

EBM involves assessing the patient, formulating a clinical question, searching for the best clinical evidence to answer the question, applying the information, and assessing the outcome. A basic question for every patient is: What is the differential diagnosis for the presenting signs and symptoms? Once the probable diagnosis is determined, further questions should arise about the best treatment, prognosis, and further diagnostic studies.

A method of formulating clinical questions is using the PICO method.

P—Patient Characteristics: What are your patient characteristics, including age, gender, and medical problems?

I—Intervention: What is your proposed intervention, drug, procedure, exposure, or diagnostic test?

C—Comparison: To what are you comparing the main intervention? (This is optional.)

O—Outcome: What outcome(s) are you looking for or measuring?

In the case of Mr. Smith:

P—45-year-old male, hypertensive, with probable migraine headaches

I—What medication would be best to add to the hydrochlorothiazide to control his blood pressure?

C—. . . compared with his self medication with ibuprofen?

O—. . . to get the best blood pressure control and help his migraines?

Once you have formulated a question, you need to choose the appropriate evidence that is accessible, timely, credible, clinically important, and applicable to the patient population. The options are paper textbooks, colleagues you work with, online reference books, journal articles, online databases, established guidelines, and critical subject reviews.

To acquire the latest medical evidence, clinicians must rely on electronic media via the Internet to search for the latest study results. Most clinicians do not have Internet access at the bedside in hospitals and clinic settings. The PDA is a tool that allows clinicians to quickly search and access evidence-based information in any clinical setting. It is portable, affordable, accessible, and easy to update. PDAs can link to Internet-connected personal computers (PCs) to download the latest information into the PDA. There are wonderful subscription services that continually update treatment and diagnostic information for the clinician so he or she reviews the latest evidence-based recommendations. The convenience of the PDA allows clinicians to review information quickly at the point of care instead of waiting until Internet access is available.

Journal watch services now can send article titles and abstracts for review from journals the clinician regularly reads. This allows the clinician to review and keep up with the exploding volume of articles when he or she has a free moment.

There now are wireless PDAs that allow instant access to the Internet and the latest published evidence using free journal search software such as PubMed, MedScape, and *Mobile* Merck*Medicus*. These are very powerful bedside tools that allow clinicians the results of the latest studies and review articles if there is wireless service available.

There are EBM products for sale, such as UptoDate, Inforetriever, BMJ Clinical Evidence, and Dynamed, that offer clinicians appraised evidence by content experts who review the latest clinical studies, write recommendations, and offer a subscription of continuous updates of common medical topics. These can be downloaded for review when there is no wireless service and are updated when you do.

Integrated PDA medical programs work with and without wireless service and offer linked drug, medical diagnostic, and treatment information with calculators, tables, drug interaction programs, and study reviews. The two reviewed in this book are Epocrates Essentials and Pepid.

It is essential that today's practicing clinicians learn how to use these tools to keep up with the rapidly growing volume of medical knowledge. Students should be taught early in their studies how to use these tools just as they learn to use their stethoscope. Faculty must become familiar with the equipment and software programs to teach the next generation of e-connected clinicians.

## Preparing for Board Examinations

Doing quick reads about common topics is excellent preparation for board examinations. There is always a little down time during breaks, at lunch time, between late patients, or commuting on public transportation when you can read up on a disease. The 5-Minute Clinical Consult (Dx in Epocrates), PEPID, *Harrison's Practice*, and the *Merck Manual* are all excellent choices for quick reads. Work your way through the table of contents concentrating on one body system at a time. You may develop a disease topic list in Documents to Go or memo pad and check off the topics as you review them. For more in-depth learning, use the PDA version of UpToDate.

## Continuing Medical Education

Practicing an EBM lifestyle promotes lifelong learning. Many of these EBM products, such as Epocrates, InfoRetriever, and UpToDate, have continuing medical education (CME ) credits for reading the content and taking a post test. Epocrates sends new topic reviews to your PDA on a timely basis; you will see the topics in the CME section of your home page. You read the article and take a multiple-choice test with instant feedback, and you are allowed to change your answer after rereading the section pertaining to the question. Your CME credits are e-mailed to you after you sync again to log the test results. This is an excellent way to keep up with the latest advances and earn CME credits for certification and licensing requirements.

Use the PDA calendar function to log the time and title of CME functions for your records. For instance, the title should begin with CME. When it's time to log your hours for professional certification on maintaining licensure, you can do a search for the letters CME and all the dates should appear from your calendar.

## Classroom Notes

As a clinical student, there are several notes, PowerPoint slide shows, and many PDF files that you would like to take with you into the clinical world as references. You can download, store, and read Microsoft Word, PowerPoint, and Adobe PDF files to an unlimited number of memory cards. Palm PDAs usually come with Documents to Go, and Adobe has its free PDF reader for PDAs available at www.adobe.com.

Students can build their own reference files from any electronic materials using the cut-and-paste feature in a Word document and use Documents to Go to transfer it to the PDA. Organizing your documents into folders and giving them a title that helps you find the information quickly is the key to managing your information.

Schools and offices may post notes on a Web site, and students can use AvantGo Web-clipping software to carry the notes on their PDAs as described in Chapter 5.

## The Future

PDAs will evolve to offer more memory, longer batteries, improved screens, better phones, and wireless integration. Wireless networks are increasing, allowing Web access in a greater number of areas. Video books showing physical examination techniques and medical and surgical procedures will be available by Web streaming or on your PDA memory card for quick review.

Video phone telemedicine using PDAs will be available to consult with specialists around the world about a patient.

It is possible that lectures for school or CME will be streamed from the Web or carried on memory cards to be viewed anytime on the PDA.

■ Interactive Learning and Testing with PDA-Web Connections

Let's consider this future scenario. You walk into your hospital to do patient rounds and all your patient data are wirelessly transmitted to your PDA. You have biometric security confirmation with a thumbprint on your PDA touch screen to identify you. You start rounds, making notes using your PDA that transfers all of your new information and orders to the hospital computers for printing, billing, and storage. As you walk out the door, all of the sensitive information is removed so you are not at risk of losing patient information once you have left the hospital grounds.

## The Future Clinician

The medical PDA of the future will be used to document patient history and physical examination, receive test results, and chart notes securely communicating with clinic and hospital computers. Coding and billing will be computed by the software and verified by the clinician.

These PDAs will allow wireless prescription generation, with a drug interaction and patient allergy check taking place even as the prescription is written. These PDAs will allow secure patient information access anywhere the clinician needs it. PDAs will be issued to all clinical students along with their new stethoscope. Software training will begin the first week of medical training.

# PDA Hardware and Software: The Basics to Begin

## Objectives

- Discuss the PDA hardware choices and options.
- Describe the nonmedical software programs bundled with most PDAs that make life a little easier and more enjoyable.

## PDA Hardware

As discussed in Chapter 1, a PDA is a personal digital assistant, a pocket electronic computer that can help provide information and communication. PDAs come with three main types of operating systems: Research in Motion (RIM) BlackBerry, Palm OS, and Microsoft Windows Mobile. There are several PDA devices in each category. Recently there has been a decline in pure PDAs and an increase in combination cell phone/PDA devices, called smart phones.

The medical software for PDAs has been dominated by Palm OS, but there is a shift to develop new programs for Windows and RIM because of their device popularity. Palm has developed a line of smart phones (Treo) using both Windows and Palm OS. There are very few medical applications for the RIM BlackBerry. It has a large share of the instant e-mail market, but because of the lack of medical options, it will not be discussed at this time. The Palm and Windows products offer instant e-mail services. Apple entered the smart phone market in 2007 with the Apple iPhone. This offers many PDA features and wireless Web browsing. Very few medical programs are available for this device at the time of this writing, so it will not be discussed as a current option. The strengths and weaknesses of each operating system, from the author's point of view, are summarized in Table 2-1.

New PDAs and smart phones are introduced to the market at a rapid pace, so this information is constantly changing and needs constant review. The key is to first choose the software that will help your daily medical practice, and then buy a PDA that will reliably run that software. There may be a size or feature that makes one PDA a better choice for you than another. Choose a PDA that will be with you at all times, because it will be the most useful. As of 2008, Palm OS has a slight advantage in the medical world because of the volume of programs available, its reliability, battery life, and cost. (Strayer & Ebell, 2005.)

A Windows Mobile PDA is a good second choice.

## How to Choose a PDA

Because PDAs and smart phones are continuously evolving with the addition of more features and capacity, some general guidelines for narrowing down your choices are presented here.

■ Comparing the Palm OS or Windows Mobile

When comparing a Palm OS or Windows Mobile (mini-Windows), make your choice based on what kinds of software you want to run. If you are used to using Windows on a desktop, you may find the Windows Mobile interface a bit more familiar because it uses similar features. You should review the available devices, check for the features

**Table 2-1** PDA and Smart Phone Operating Systems

| PDA | RIM BlackBerry | Windows Mobile | Palm OS | Apple Mac OS |
|---|---|---|---|---|
| **Market Share** | Large | Large | Moderate | Small |
| **Medical Applications** | Small | Moderate | Large | Small |
| **Cost** | Moderate | Moderate | Moderate | Moderate |

Strayer, S, Reynolds, P, Ebell, M. *Handhelds in Medicine, a Practical Guide for Clinicians.* New York: Springer; 2005, pp 3–5.

you want, and visit a store where you can see, feel, and play with the device. A listing of the latest Palm OS PDAs is available at www.palm.com, and the latest Windows Mobile devices can be viewed at www.microsoft.com/windowsmobile/devices/default.mspx.

### ■ Memory

Sufficient memory is critical; without it, the number of applications that can be added to your device is limited. Generally, PDAs come with 32 to 128 MB of memory. Much more important than the amount of memory that comes with the device, however, is whether you can add more. Virtually all devices (with the exception of very low-end models) now accept memory expansion cards. These cards are commonly available in a number of sizes, from 128 MB to 4 GB, providing almost unlimited storage capacity for PDAs. Programs installed on memory cards may run slower than those stored in the handheld, so it might be wise to store programs used less frequently on the memory card.

### ■ Software

The real power of handheld devices comes from the software applications you are able to add. Palm has been in the PDA market longer and there are more medical programs available. The software library for Windows Mobile is improving and many popular applications originally written for the Palm OS now have a Windows counterpart. An excellent guide for choosing the right software is available at the Americal Medical Student Association Web site at www.amsa.org/meded/choosingapda.cfm.

### ■ Size

Size does matter when it comes to selecting a PDA. If the device is too big or heavy to have it with you at all times, it will be of very little use, regardless of how many features it has. Having the PDA clipped on using a belt clip makes it instantly accessible and prevents loss. If you have a coat with pockets, your PDA can fit next to your stethoscope (but find a way to clip it in to prevent fatal falls). Historically, Palm OS–based devices tend to be more compact, but as new generations of devices appear, PDA manufacturers consistently are introducing smaller and sleeker handheld models. The smart phones are larger and heavier than regular cell phones. Go to a store that has several models to look at, feel, and play with.

## ■ Battery Life

As has always been the case with portable computing, a device is only good if it has the power to run. Adding functionality such as color screens, Bluetooth, and wireless connectivity increases the power demands and frequency with which devices must be recharged. It is best to turn off wireless features when not in use to save battery power. If you are in your vehicle frequently, auto adapter chargers will help to keep your PDA recharged.

## ■ Data Input

PDAs use a stylus for data input on the screen, using a shorthand character recognition program called Graffitti, or a screen keyboard for direct entry of letters and numbers. Many new PDAs have a small button-style keyboard. Most devices now support larger detachable keyboards that can be used for data entry. Some may fold for portability. These add-ons have a wide range in price but can dramatically increase the speed of data entry. It is recommended that you use your PC to do large amounts of text entry and send it to your PDA for reference. If you work around bar code systems, there are PDAs with built-in bar code readers for scanning patient arm bands, medication packages, or items on the patient chart.

## ■ Functionality

Both Windows Mobile and Palm OS devices have options such as voice-recording capability for dictation or voice memos, MP3 audio players for music, global positioning system (GPS) for instant directions, and video players for watching TV shows or instructional video clips. The choice of PDA may depend on the extra features you find most useful in your daily life. You can truly have one device that does it all, instead of having a digital music player, a separate GPS device, and a separate voice recorder. The more features in the PDA, the larger the size and greater the weight. It is wise to travel to the nearest store where you can see and feel the PDA in action to decide whether it is functional for you. If your PDA is too big or bulky to have with you at all times, it will be inconvenient to use for medical reference.

■ Expandability

Expansion slots allow you to add things like memory cards and other accessories. All current PDAs use a small, removable, secure digital (SD) memory card that can store from 128 MB to 4 GB of data. These cards are the same and also fit into many digital cameras for picture storage. A 2-GB card can store the equivalent of 100 large (20 MB) medical textbooks with pictures. Find out the maximum your PDA will recognize. You'll want to get one or more of these memory cards to store the reference books you'd like to have at your fingertips. Memory cards also allow you to store music, pictures, and even video files. You can have all your applications on one card or have a card for each application; for instance, one card for medical information, another for music, and yet another for pictures.

■ Price

PDAs range widely in price with physical size, memory, and phone/wireless features being the most influential factors in pricing. Smart phones may be cheaper when you buy them with a contract for cell phone service. The best way to research pricing is to choose the cell phone provider with the best features and coverage for you, and then look at the smart phone options. Go to the cell phone store and look at the devices available.

■ To Phone or Not to Phone

Throw away your pager and cell phone because now you can do it all with one device. There are cell phone PDAs that have all of these features; they actually will dial the number in your phone book, log onto the Internet, get your e-mail, and allow real-time Web surfing. You should choose your cell phone service with the best coverage and price first, then see what models of PDA phones they offer. Most companies will offer the PDA phone at a discount if you sign a 1- or 2-year contract. Choose the model that appeals to you and best meets your needs. If you want to get e-mail and Internet service on your PDA phone, there usually is a data charge per minute or a monthly charge for unlimited service. Many universities and health care systems have discount contracts with a cell service vendor, so start there for the best price.

PDA phones usually are equipped with Bluetooth to allow wireless headsets for hands-free phone conversations and can link to new automobiles in which the Bluetooth system is embedded. This is a safety feature to keep the driver's eyes on the road when driving.

Choosing the PDA phone option may be the best way to ensure that your PDA is always with you so you can practice EBM lookups throughout your workday. A PDA in your locker, purse, or office desk will not allow you to do frequent bedside lookups.

### ■ Beaming

The PDA usually has an infrared beaming port (IrDA, which works much like a TV remote control) to send and receive information from another PDA. There may be compatibility issues if the PDAs do not have the same operating system (for example, Palm OS versus Windows). This feature allows you to share text files, pictures, programs that are not locked, contacts, and calendars. Instead of swapping business cards with colleagues, you can beam your electronic card to their PDA from yours in a second. You can transmit information to PCs and printers if they have infrared ports.

### ■ Bluetooth Versus Wi-Fi

Bluetooth is a close-range wireless system that allows wireless transmission between your PDA and other devices that have Bluetooth capability. The usual distance is 30 feet or less, and it provides a wireless, point-to-point communication for PDAs, laptop PCs, printers, mobile phones, audio components, and other devices. This capability would allow you to sync your PDA to your Bluetooth-enabled laptop or PC.

Wi-fi is short for wireless fidelity and represents high-speed access to the Internet or local area networks. Wi-fi connections can be made up to about 300 feet away from a hot spot (slang for a wi-fi networking node). When your PDA has a wi-fi networking card or built-in chip, you can look at the Internet wirelessly. A wi-fi SD card can be purchased that has both extra memory and adds wireless connectivity.

This card fits in the SD memory slot of the PDA and sticks out about an inch. This, however, may not be compatible with all PDA models.

## Best PDA Recommendation for EBM

The EBM-PDA should be able to connect to the Internet through wireless networks or cell service to acquire the latest medical evidence at the bedside.

The best EBM-PDA is the one you will keep on your person at all times when you are seeing patients and the one you will use to do quick lookups at the point of care. This will not work if your PDA is locked in your desk, purse, locker, car, or home. The entire reason to develop an EBM lifestyle in your daily routine is to have the information at your fingertips for quick reference. Choose the device with the features and software combinations that will make it an indispensable tool that you'll have with you at all times.

## Programs that Come with the PDA

The built-in basic functions of all PDAs include an address and phone number book, a memo pad, a calculator, a to-do list, a schedule with alarms and reminders, and a way to link data to and from your base computer. You can use the address book for all of your contacts, both professional and personal. The schedule keeps you on time and helps you plan appointments, lectures, and even patient visits. An excellent online tutorial on using the basic PDA functions is available at www. doctorsgadgets.com/the-doctors-pda-and-smartphone-handbook/. Video demonstrations of the common programs and features, labeled Video 2–1 and Video 2–2, are available on the CD-ROM.

■ Sync Software

All PDAs come with software that allows communication with a PC; in other words, to synchronize, hence the name sync software. This is critical for backups and getting updated information and programs from your PC to your PDA. You should have Web access on your PC to download the programs reviewed in this book. You should get in the habit of syncing to your PC at least once a week. If you ever need to restore the programs and information on your PDA, it will only be as current as the last time you synced.

■ Reset

All PDAs have a button to do a soft reset, which is the equivalent of the Ctrl-Alt-Del combination to reset a PC that becomes unruly. This is useful to do if your PDA becomes unresponsive while using an application. There is a procedure and combination of keys to do a hard reset if the soft one does not work. This usually will erase all the data stored on your PDA and restore the factory settings. If you need to do this, you should be able to restore all of your information as of your last sync.

■ Security

All PDAs have a method of applying an owner password when they start, and they allow you to block viewing of private files. If you plan to carry patient information on your PDA, you will need to have HIPAA-compliant security enabled to protect privacy. The PDA is a wonderful reference tool for EBM, but it can be a security issue if you choose to store patient information. The other security issue is storing sensitive personal information that you may wish to protect.

■ Contacts

The contact manager is an electronic address book to store names, phone numbers, e-mails, addresses, pictures, notes, and category. This is most helpful so that you have your medical contacts or consultants all together for easy lookup. You can separate your personal contacts from others by assigning each person a category. If you are a user of Microsoft Outlook, you can link your PDA list with your PC. If you have a PDA phone, you can use your contact list as your phone book and click on a name to contact them.

■ Appointments

The appointment book allows you to plan your time with work schedule, on-call time, appointments, classes, conferences, meetings, and personal reminders. It can be used to track your continuing medical education (CME) hours when you attend meetings. You can make appointments with a reminder alarm to keep you on time. It is easy to set up recurring appointments and block out entire days for vacations and holidays.

■ To-Do List

If you have tasks you want to prioritize and track, the to-do list is a wonderful tool to use as a reminder and record of accomplishments. Tasks can be categorized into personal, medical, or anything you set. You can set the task priority as 1, 2, 3, and so forth, and even add a note about the task.

■ Calculator

A standard calculator for routine math problems is included in each PDA. In addition, there are medical calculators, with built-in clinical calculations, that can be added into the applications reviewed in this book.

■ Link with Microsoft Documents

Palm PDAs usually come with a program called Documents to Go, which allows you to transfer and edit Microsoft Word, Excel, and Power-Point files on your PDA. The Windows Mobile PDAs do this seamlessly. This allows you to build your own references using notes from class handouts or meeting notes. You can use the cut-and-paste function of Word to clip text from Web sites or e-text books and store the information as a PDA reference. You can include pictures, graphs, and calculations just like your PC documents. These files can be stored on your memory card to save internal memory.

■ Adobe PDF Documents

Adobe offers a free PDF reader, allowing you to transfer, store, and read Adobe PDF files on your PDA. This allows you to view text and pictures as well. These files can be stored on your memory card to save internal memory. This PDF reader is available at www.adobe.com.

■ E-mail

The Palm PDA has an e-mail program called VersaMail that can be configured to download your business or personal e-mail. The wireless PDAs will need to be in a wireless area, but the cell phone–connected PDA can link anywhere there is cell service. The e-mail allows you to set preferences to remove deleted e-mails from your e-mail server and add attachments. Both Windows and Palm PDAs can be set up to connect to Microsoft Outlook e-mail services. This allows you to download and carry your contact lists, schedule, and e-mail.

### ■ Web Viewing

Both Palm and Windows PDAs provide a Web browser that allows Web site viewing on your PDA while in a wireless environment or a cell-supplied area, depending on your carrier. The trick is viewing large Web pages with a great number of images on a small PDA screen. There are many PDA-friendly Web sites that have text formatted for the PDA screen and few images. You can choose to turn images off to increase the download and viewing speed.

### ■ Web Clipping

There are free programs that allow Web clipping, the downloading of Web pages when you are linked to an Internet-connected PC, a wireless PDA in a wireless environment, or a cellular PDA on the data network. One advantage to Web clipping is being able to copy Web content to your PDA for reading and reference later when you may not have Web access. Web clipping also allows you to create your own e-books from Web pages that are updated the next time you sync to a Web-connected PC or when you have wireless access.

### ■ Business Expenses

For ease of accounting purposes, there is a business expense tracker to track travel, food, parking, and other travel expenses for taxes or reimbursement.

### ■ Picture Viewer

Many PDAs have built-in cameras that can take digital pictures and small movie clips. The pictures usually are stored in j-peg (.jpg) format which is standard for sharing, printing, and e-mailing. Picture and movie files use a large amount of memory, so you need a memory card to store these files. For medical uses, the camera can be used to document rashes, lesions, or other patient education pictures.

Any picture you can scan into a .jpg format can be sent to your PDA memory card for use in teaching. Some digital cameras use the same SD memory card as the PDAs, and you can view your pictures right from the camera by inserting the camera's SD memory card into the PDA memory slot.

■ Audio Player

The audio player allows you to enjoy stereo music or listen to medical lectures. Some PDAs allow digital audio recording for dictation. Audio files take up a great deal of memory, so an additional memory card is a must.

Most PDAs now have music-playing software. Palm has a PDA version of Real Player, and Windows PDAs have the Windows Media Player. You can store hours of music from your CD collection to your memory card for your listening pleasure. PDAs have a stereo headphone jack, and the Palm Treos need a small stereo adapter for private listening.

■ Video Players

With memory storage increasing and the ability to compress video getting better each year, you can convert DVDs and video files to 1 MB-per-minute video files. (A 2-GB card could store 200 minutes of compressed video.) The screen is small but the portable entertainment and education factor is huge.

The newest generation of PDA phones and wireless PDAs offer streaming video capability, which allows you to watch the same video you can view on your Internet-connected PC. This allows TV access and movies on demand. The ability to have medical training videos about procedure and surgical techniques, interviewing skills, and continuing medical education is very near.

■ Medical Applications Using the Standard Programs

Standard software can be used to do medical tasks. Use the memo feature or Word document reader to copy reference documents to your PDA. For instance, you may have a list of common ICD-9 diagnosis codes in a Word file. Convert it for your PDA and download it to your PDA as a PDF, Word file, or memo file. You can do the same with drug lists, contact lists, differential diagnosis, and guidelines. Use the phone book to keep a list of your consultant and hospital phone numbers. These can be separated by category types.

A spreadsheet like Excel can be used by students to log procedures using current procedural terminology (CPT) codes and evaluation/management E/M codes for credentialing and clinical rotation documentation. There are commercial software PDA-to-Web programs that are designed do this as well.

■ Organizing Your Applications

The PDA allows you to organize your applications into categories to rapidly find the correct icon to tap. You can make a new category such as "medical" to place all your medical application icons on one screen.

# Differential Diagnosis and Physical Examination Tools for PDAs

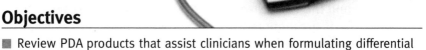

## Objectives

- Review PDA products that assist clinicians when formulating differential diagnosis.
- Review PDA resources that provide medical history and physical examination references.

## One Sees What One Knows

There are no evidence-based medicine resources that will help an incorrect diagnosis to guide the medical workup. Differential diagnosis, or the prioritized list of possible patient diagnosis, is the critical first step to lead into excellent evidence-based care.

Differential diagnosis is the heart of medicine, guiding the clinician's history, physical exam, and testing. As the German author and scientist Johann Wolfgang von Goethe (1798) elegantly stated: "One sees what one knows." Clinicians will integrate and explore patient signs and symptoms only from their knowledge base of potential diagnosis possibilities. This knowledge base of differential diagnosis grows with clinical experience and reading, but students need a reference list from which to start and every seasoned clinician needs a reminder now and then.

A clinician should have a working differential diagnosis list with every patient's new presenting problem. This differential will narrow from a long list to a few top contenders based on integrating the patient's history, physical exam findings, and laboratory and radiology results. The more experienced the clinician, the quicker the signs and symptoms point to specific diagnosis. The proper differential will keep the clinician efficient, cost effective, and help prevent him or her from missing critical conditions. Clinicians should be pessimistic optimists, considering what diagnostic possibilities can cause serious harm but not alarm the patient.

Students beginning their journey into clinical medicine often are assigned patient workups not knowing the chief complaint; are not aware of the problem-oriented approach to the history, physical examination, or diagnostic studies; and have not learned all the possible problems needed to formulate a differential diagnosis. A quick reference allows the student to start the patient interview, hear the chief complaint, excuse themselves from the room, and do a quick review of the differential diagnosis. This allows a return to the patient with a focused plan to narrow the hunt for the diagnosis.

Clinicians should listen and facilitate getting the patient's chief complaint (CC) and the seven aspects of the history of the present illness (HPI). The CC is the main reason the patient came seeking care, with the duration of the symptoms or signs. The HPI should follow and include as much of the seven aspects as applicable. A mnemonic that can help the clinician remember these seven aspects is LOCATES:

L—Location and radiation

O—Other associated symptoms related to the CC

C—Character of the CC

A—Aggravating and alleviating factors; what makes it better or worse

T—Timing: the duration, constant versus intermittent

E—Environment, or the setting where the CC occurs

S—Severity of the CC on a numeric scale where zero is none and 10 is the worst ever

These seven aspects work well for pain as a CC, but may not fit other complaints.

Once the CC and HPI are obtained, a differential diagnosis should be formulated and a focused history and physical examination performed. The differential diagnosis is the road map for the rest of the clinical encounter, so it needs to be accurate and well thought out.

Seasoned clinicians know from experience what is common, what is dangerous, and what combination of symptoms may point to a disease presentation. The student does not yet have these filtering skills and rapid references are needed. There are five products that will be reviewed as this doorway to the correct diagnosis and evidence-based treatment.

## Differential Diagnosis Mnemonics

One approach to learn complex differential lists is to use memory tools like mnemonics. There is a free Palm OS program by Allan Platt (2000) called *Differential Diagnosis Mnemonics and the Medical History.* This was first published as a pocket-sized booklet and it has been adapted to a Palm OS application by Emory medical student Michael Ward. This program is text based and has an alphabetical list of 64 common presenting patient complaints. This product is free at www.EmoryPA.org.

There is a mnemonic for each part of the medical history and common problems; for example: you are seeing a 20-year-old male with 2 days of yellow sclera (jaundice), nausea, and right upper quadrant abdominal pain. You want to refresh your differential diagnosis of jaundice using *Differential Diagnosis Mnemonics* on your PDA. You will enter the program through the title screen and see a Table of Contents with all of the symptoms and corresponding mnemonics. Tap on the symptom to see the full differential diagnosis. A video demonstration of *Differential Diagnosis Mnemonics*, labeled Video 3–1, is available on the CD-ROM.

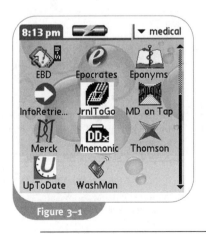

Choose DDx with the doctor's bag icon.

Figure 3–1

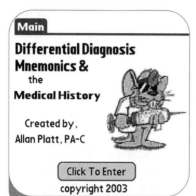

**Main**

# Differential Diagnosis Mnemonics &
the
**Medical History**

Created by,
Allan Platt, PA-C

[ Click To Enter ]

copyright 2003

Figure 3-2

This is the opening screen for the program. Tap the Click To Enter box to see the next screen.

---

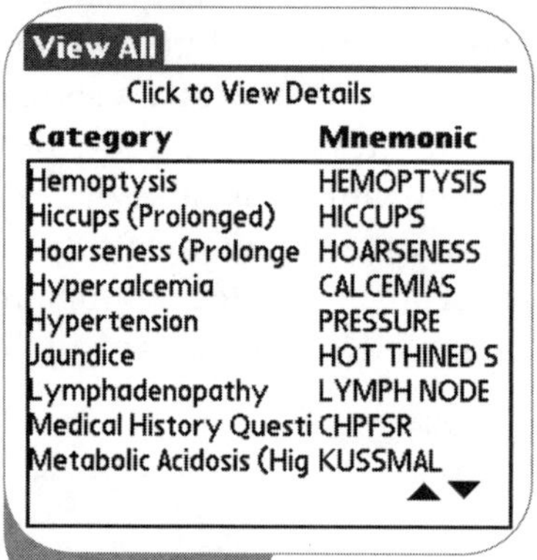

**View All**

Click to View Details

| Category | Mnemonic |
|----------|----------|
| Hemoptysis | HEMOPTYSIS |
| Hiccups (Prolonged) | HICCUPS |
| Hoarseness (Prolonge | HOARSENESS |
| Hypercalcemia | CALCEMIAS |
| Hypertension | PRESSURE |
| Jaundice | HOT THINED S |
| Lymphadenopathy | LYMPH NODE |
| Medical History Questi | CHPFSR |
| Metabolic Acidosis (Hig | KUSSMAL |

▲▼

Figure 3-3

Scroll down the alphabetical list to Jaundice. Tap on Jaundice to see the differential diagnosis for the mnemonic HOT THINED SAP.

---

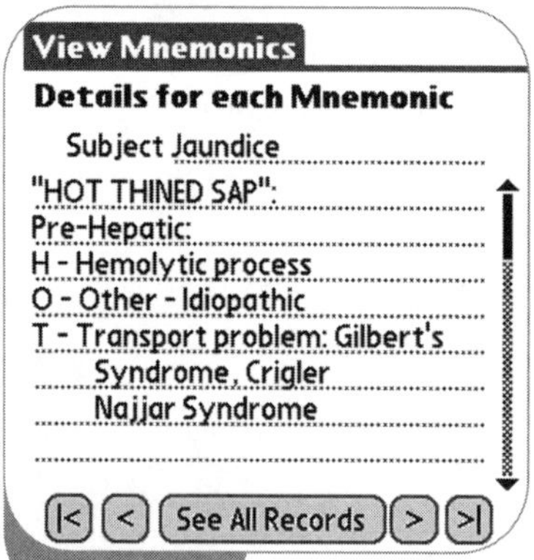

**View Mnemonics**

**Details for each Mnemonic**

Subject Jaundice

"HOT THINED SAP":
Pre-Hepatic:
H - Hemolytic process
O - Other - Idiopathic
T - Transport problem: Gilbert's
        Syndrome, Crigler
        Najjar Syndrome

[|<] [<] [ See All Records ] [>] [>|]

Figure 3-4

Scrolling down, you would see:

Liver Causes:
T—Toxin: Alcohol, carbon tetrachloride
H—Hereditary: Dubin Johnson or Roter syndrome
I— Infection: Viral—A, B, C, D, E, mono, CMV, toxoplasmosis, syphilis, ameba
N—Neoplasm: Hepatoma, metastatic cancer
E—End-stage liver disease: cirrhosis
D—Drugs: INH, halothane, estrogens, NSAIDS, acetaminophen, PTU, sulfas

Postliver Causes:
S—Stones: Gall stones, sclerosing cholangitis
A—Atresia of the bile duct
P—Pancreatic neoplasm or inflammation

---

# Diagnosaurus

A free program available from McGraw-Hill for Palm OS and Pocket PC is *Diagnosaurus,* an electronic book by Dr. Roni F. Zeiger. It is available at http://books.mcgraw-hill.com/medical/diagnosaurus/index. html. The PDA book reader is supplied by Unbound Medicine, the supplier of other McGraw-Hill PDA textbooks and the free Merck *Medicus* PDA program reviewed in Chapter 6.

This text-based reference program has a thousand-plus differential diagnoses that can be searched by disease, symptom, or organ system. There is a medicine and a surgery list, and the differential diagnoses are listed in order of prevalence. There are "not-to-be-missed" listings to alert the clinician to potentially serious conditions to consider.

The following screen shots show how to start the *Diagnosaurus* program. Then, using the same patient example, they show how to look up the differential diagnosis of jaundice. A video demonstration of *Diagnosaurus,* labeled Video 3–2, is available on the CD-ROM.

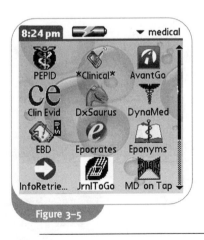

Figure 3–5

Tap on the DxSaurus dinosaur icon to start the program.

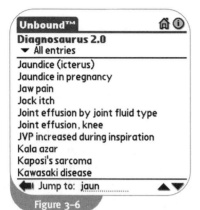

Figure 3-6

Tap in the letters "jaun" in the Jump to: space at the bottom and the list will scroll to the diseases beginning with "j".

Tap Jaundice (icterus).

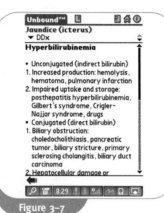

Figure 3-7

This figure shows the differential diagnosis of jaundice or hyperbilirubinemia. It is divided by unconjugated, then conjugated bilirubin.

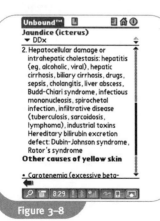

Figure 3-8

The hepatic causes are listed under the biliary causes and then other causes of yellow skin.

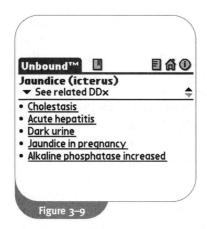

Tap on the drop-down box under the title Jaundice (icterus) and tap "See related DDx" to get the list shown here that may guide you to other related lists.

Figure 3–9

## Epocrates Sx: Differential Diagnosis Using Multiple Signs and Symptoms

The Sx program in Epocrates began at the Laboratory of Computer Science of the Department of Medicine at Massachusetts General Hospital. The computer staff developed a differential diagnosis assistant computer program called DXplain in 1984. This program allowed the user to enter patient signs and symptoms and would compute the most likely diagnosis based on a mathematical algorithm. National distribution of DXplain with a database of approximately 2000 diseases began in 1987 over the dial-up AMANET. After AMANET ceased operation in 1990, DXplain continued to be distributed over dial-up networks until 1995. Between 1991 and 1996, DXplain was available as a stand-alone version that could be loaded on an individual PC. Since 1996, it has been available as a Web-based application.

The current DXplain knowledge base includes over 2200 diseases and over 4900 clinical findings (symptoms, signs, epidemiologic data and laboratory, endoscopic and radiologic findings). The average disease description includes 53 findings (with a range of 10 to over 100). Each disease/finding pair has two numbers describing the relationship: one representing the frequency with which the finding occurs in the disease and the other the degree to which the presence of the finding suggests consideration of the disease. There are over 230,000 individual data points in the database representing disease/finding relationships. In addition, each finding has an associated disease-independent importance attribute from 1 to 5, indicating how important it is to explain the presence of the finding. Each disease also has two associated values: one that is a crude approximation of its prevalence (very common, common, rare, or very rare) and the other of its importance (ranked between 1 and 5) and intended to reflect the impact of not considering the disease if it is present.

In January of 2006, Epocrates partnered with the developers of DXplain and the developers of *Griffith's 5-Minute Clinical Consult* to produce a PDA version called Epocrates SxDx. This is a unique integrated "smart" differential diagnosis generator linked with a current evidence-based, continually updated medical textbook with 1200 diseases, conditions, and clinical topics. It allows the user to input several signs and symptoms and it computes the most likely diagnosis. The integrated product reviewed in the next chapter is Epocrates Essentials.

Clinicians at the bedside or exam table can enter on Epocrates Sx the patient's age, gender, duration of symptoms, and any number of symptoms, physical exam findings, lab or radiology results, and the most likely differential diagnosis will display in descending order of prevalence. There is a "refine" function that asks further questions to clarify and a "rare" function to see a list of less-common diseases that may present with the entered list. All of the diseases are linked to the Dx program for a full description of basic information, diagnostic confirmation, signs and symptoms, lab and radiology findings, and treatment. Disease ICD-9 codes are even listed for coding.

The following screens will demonstrate how to use Epocrates Sx to generate a differential diagnosis for a 20-year-old male with 2 days of yellow sclera (jaundice), nausea, and right upper quadrant abdominal pain. A video demonstration of Epocrates Sx, labeled Video 3–3, is available on the CD-ROM.

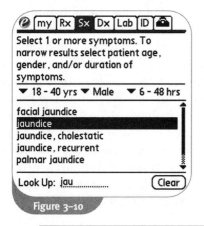

Figure 3–10

Using the previous patient example, open Epocrates Sx and enter the patient's age range, gender, and symptom duration using drop-down boxes. Then enter the symptoms jaundice and nausea in the lookup box. Tap the text in the list to add them.

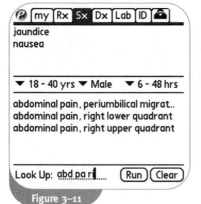

Figure 3-11

You can enter the first few letters of the words you want with spaces in between to speed the lookup. Type in "abd pa ri" (see the bottom of the figure) to get the list given. Select abdominal pain, right upper quadrant/enter, then Run.

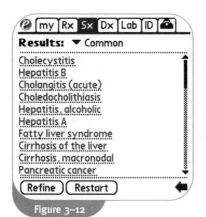

Figure 3-12

After a few seconds, the program will respond with a differential diagnosis list. Clicking on the Refine button (shown at the bottom) will give a checklist asking if the following are present from your physical exam or lab findings: Cholecystitis, Hepatitis B, Cholangitis (acute), and so forth. Tap the Refine button to see the screen in Figure 3-13.

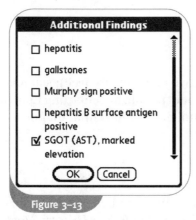

Figure 3-13

The Refine screen lists additional signs and symptoms you may consider. If you know that the SGOT/AST is elevated, check the box and tap the OK button.

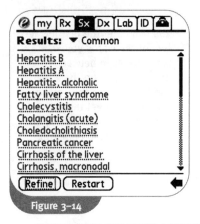

This screen shows the differential list with Hepatitis B and A and Hepatitis, alcoholic to be the three top contenders. You can link to the Dx text for any of those diagnoses by using the Dx tab at the top of the screen and reading a capsule summary in the 5-Minute Clinical Consult.

Tap on the Common drop-down box and then tap Rare for a list of rare causes (see Figure 3-15).

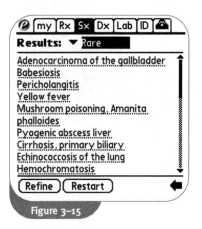

This list is good to review and keep in the back of your mind if the common things do not pan out.

Check out all three programs (two of which are free); schools and large groups often can arrange discount pricing by contacting Epocrates. With these PDA programs, the clinician's differential diagnosis can expand as knowledge increases.

## Clinical Methods

There are very few physical examination–medical history reference books for the PDA. However, *Clinical Methods: The History, The Phys-*

*ical, and Laboratory Examinations, Third Edition,* is a free comprehensive full textbook available as a download at www.ncbi.nlm.nih.gov/books/bookres.fcgi/cm/pda.html and requires the free Mobipocket reader to be installed on your PDA. This textbook appeared in print in 1990, but the aspects of the history and physical examination have not changed much in the past 20 years. This is a timeless classic that is a ready reference for students and seasoned clinicians. There are illustrations and some differential diagnoses.

The following screen shots show *Clinical Methods* on the PDA after starting the MobiPocket Reader from the main menu. A video demonstration of *Clinical Methods*, labeled Video 3–4, is available on the CD-ROM.

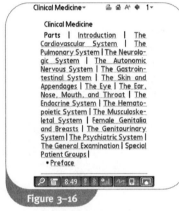

Figure 3–16

This screen shows the table of contents listing the body systems in the book.

The house icon will take you to the table of contents. The back arrow (also at the top) will take you to last page viewed. The number-down arrow allows you to jump to any page. The folder icon will leave this book and list all of your Mobipocket books.

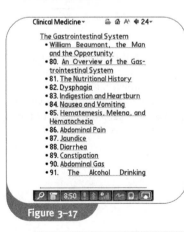

Figure 3–17

Tapping on The Gastrointestinal System reveals the following submenu of GI topics. Tap on Jaundice.

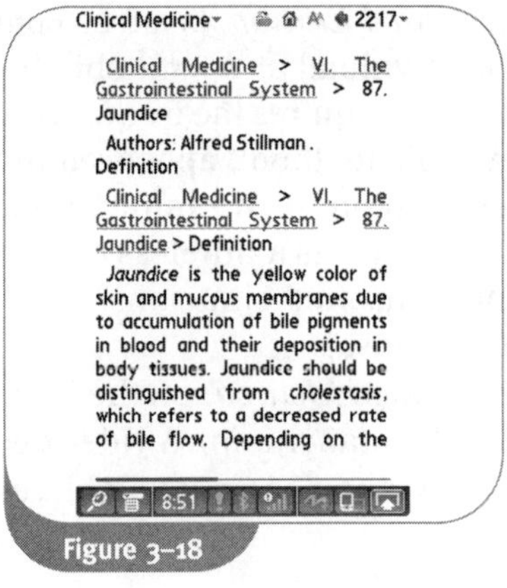

Clinical Medicine > VI. The Gastrointestinal System > 87. Jaundice

Authors: Alfred Stillman .
Definition

Clinical Medicine > VI. The Gastrointestinal System > 87. Jaundice > Definition

*Jaundice* is the yellow color of skin and mucous membranes due to accumulation of bile pigments in blood and their deposition in body tissues. Jaundice should be distinguished from *cholestasis*, which refers to a decreased rate of bile flow. Depending on the

🔍 📄 8:51 ⋮ ⋮ °⋮ 〜 ▯ 🖼

**Figure 3–18**

Tapping on Jaundice opened this screen. This is the first page of text describing jaundice. Tapping anywhere on the screen will scroll the page down to the next screen of text.

---

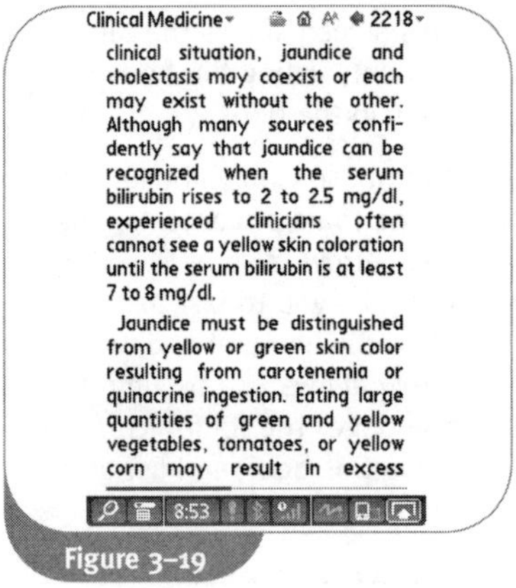

clinical situation, jaundice and cholestasis may coexist or each may exist without the other. Although many sources confidently say that jaundice can be recognized when the serum bilirubin rises to 2 to 2.5 mg/dl, experienced clinicians often cannot see a yellow skin coloration until the serum bilirubin is at least 7 to 8 mg/dl.

Jaundice must be distinguished from yellow or green skin color resulting from carotenemia or quinacrine ingestion. Eating large quantities of green and yellow vegetables, tomatoes, or yellow corn may result in excess

🔍 📄 8:53 ⋮ ⋮ °⋮ 〜 ▯ 🖼

**Figure 3–19**

This screen shows the reference text for jaundice with background information, differential diagnosis, and physical examination considerations.

---

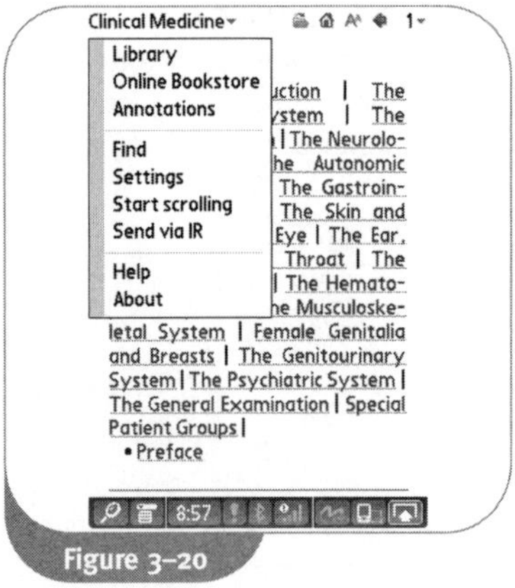

Library
Online Bookstore   uction  |   The
Annotations        ystem  |   The
                   | The Neurolo-
Find               he Autonomic
Settings           The Gastroin-
Start scrolling    The Skin and
Send via IR        Eye | The Ear,
                   Throat | The
Help               | The Hemato-
About              he Musculoske-
letal System | Female Genitalia and Breasts | The Genitourinary System | The Psychiatric System | The General Examination | Special Patient Groups |
    • Preface

🔍 📄 8:57 ⋮ ⋮ °⋮ 〜 ▯ 🖼

**Figure 3–20**

Tap on the book title at the top of the screen and this drop-down menu appears. There is a find option in which you can search the text of the entire book.

---

# Internet Web Reference: *Bedside Diagnosis*

*Bedside Diagnosis* is a free Web book with evidence to support the techniques of the physical examination posted on the Internet by the American College of Physicians (ACP) at www.acponline.org/clinical_information/resources/bedside/. This site can be accessed by a Web-connected PDA or captured as a Web book using AvantGo as discussed in Chapter 5. This is a good EBM resource to use when teaching physical examination skills.

The following screen shots show how *Bedside Diagnosis* should appear on a Palm PDA Web browser when looking up a physical exam technique called "auscultatory percussion of the liver." A video demonstration of *Bedside Diagnosis*, labeled Video 3–5, is available on the CD-ROM.

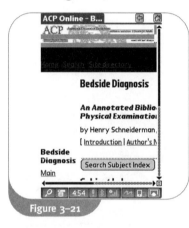

Figure 3–21

Using your PDA Web browser, go to the *Bedside Diagnosis* Web site. This is the home page in the PDA Blazer browser. This Web site is designed for PC screens and will not fit on the small PDA screen. You must use the horizontal and vertical scroll bars to navigate the screen.

Note the Search text box toward the top of the opening screen that allows you to enter a search term, or you may want to browse by topics. If you are interested in "Auscultatory percussion of the liver," enter AUS above the Search Subject Index button and then hit the Search button.

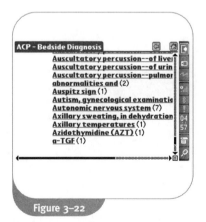

Figure 3–22

An alphabetical list of topics appears. Tap on Auscultatory percussion—of liver, and the references would be listed in a new screen.

# Integrated EBM Programs

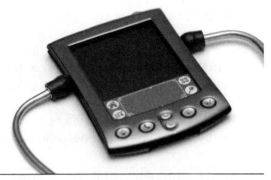

## Objectives

■ Discuss the advantages of integrated medical programs that have interlinked topics covering differential diagnosis, disease reference, lab values, drug reference, infectious disease, medical calculators, ICD-9, codes, and guidelines.

■ Review two integrated programs, Epocrates Essentials and PEPID, using a case-based approach to compare them.

## What Is an Integrated Program?

Many PDA programs and references perform a single task like providing drug information, differential diagnosis, infection treatment guides, and medical references. The best software tools for busy clinicians bundle the best of these tools and integrate them to work together for speed and efficiency. Currently, there are two programs that are the leaders in this category: Epocrates Essentials and PEPID. Skyscape and Unbound Medicine have released bundled book products called Constellation and Medicine Central. They do not meet the criteria for integrated software and they will be discussed in the PDA chapter. This chapter will review the features of Epocrates and PEPID and use a case-based approach to demonstrate how they work.

Because of the wealth of quick information these two programs offer, they encourage clinicians to use them at the point of care. This allows instant review and learning as the day goes by. By offering the best and most common PDA functions bundled together, these products are highly recommended for all clinicians. There are many similarities between the two products and many unique features that may make one work better for you. If PDA memory and budget permit, having both products may be an alternative to choosing one over the other.

It is the author's recommendation that all students and practicing clinicians should get Epocrates Essentials. Students may wish to order the additional medical dictionary for an extra fee. All students doing an emergency department rotation should download and use the free 1-month PEPID trial. All practicing clinicians who do any emergency or intensive care work should do the free 1-month PEPID trial and strongly consider purchasing it.

Table 4-1 details the differences between the two programs using information found at www.epocrates.com and www.pepid.com.

**Table 4-1** Differences and Similarities between Epocrates Essentials and PEPID

| Feature | Epocrates Essentials | PEPID |
|---|---|---|
| Platform | Palm/Win/RIM | Palm/Win/RIM |
| Design | Integrated programs | All one program |
| Space (Palm OS) PDA/memory card | 5MB/5.7MB | 4 MB/13 MB |
| Student-group discount | Yes, call | Yes, call |
| Free trial | Some, such as Rx, CME, tables | Yes, 30 days |
| Differential diagnosis | Sx; enter multiple signs and symptoms; one of the best differential diagnosis programs available | Minimal; must know disease and then look up |
| Lab guide | Included, linked to disease and includes ICD-9 | Extra fee; 300 tests |
| Disease description | 5 min cc 1200 diseases, Dx | 2700 topics by PEPID authors; more details with 400 EBM recommendations |

**Table 4-1** Differences and Similarities between Epocrates Essentials and PEPID (continued)

| Feature | Epocrates Essentials | PEPID |
|---|---|---|
| Non-Rx–alternative treatment | Included, Rx | Included |
| Rx treatment | Included, 3000 drugs | Included, more extensive—6500 |
| Rx interactions IV and PO | Included | Included |
| Infectious disease tool | Included, drug by bug or infection body site | None |
| Formulary and Medicare part D | Included | None |
| Prevention | Included | None |
| EBM links | Mobile CME, must look up topic InfoPOEMs | Built in EBM, reviews in some subjects |
| ICD-9 codes | Easy to access within each disease in Dx and in lab | Hard to find, must look up special list and know body system category |
| Dictionary | Add on *Stedman's* for minimal fee | Built in |
| Med calculator | 30 formulas | 3000 formulas |
| CME | Included Cat 1 AMA | None |

## A Case to Solve

A 32-year-old female bank financial analyst presents to the emergency department with 6 hours of right-sided pleuritic chest pain and shortness of breath. The pain began suddenly in the morning while she was getting dressed for work. She has had no tenderness in her legs and no pedal edema. She has not had any fever or chills, cough, hemoptysis, night sweats, or unexplained weight loss. She has no prior medical problems or hospitalizations, and she does not smoke, drink alcohol, or use street drugs. She takes oral contraceptives and an occasional acetaminophen for headaches. She is taking the supplement echinacea to help her nasal congestion symptoms.

Physical exam reveals a thin female in some discomfort: Pulse 105, Respirations 20, BP 130/90, pulse oximetry 96 percent. Chest/lung exam is normal with no chest wall tenderness, no wheezing or decreased breath sounds. Cardiac exam is normal.

■ What is the differential diagnosis?
■ What is the appropriate workup?
■ What ICD-9 diagnosis code do you use on the lab slips?
■ What are the best treatment options?

## Epocrates Essentials

Epocrates Essentials is an integrated group of medical reference products, all inter-linked so the user does not have to leave one reference to enter another. It combines the Sx differential diagnosis program demonstrated in Chapter 3 with Dx, the 5-Minute Clinical Consult disease reference book. Also included is the Rx drug reference including CAM therapies, a drug-drug interaction program, dosage calculator, health plan formularies with copay, coverage and prior authorization information (including the only place to currently get Medicare D formulary information on the PDA), DocAlert clinical messaging (relevant, timely clinical and specialty news from the FDA, CDC, and other groups), MedMath clinical calculator, and the MobileCME learning system with current evidence-based medical topics in your specialty. The Essentials program includes a lab reference with differential diagnosis for abnormal values linked to Dx, which is an infectious disease program labeled ID that allows review by infection body system, organism, or drug, and Tables, a multitude of reference materials including guidelines for ACLS, PALS, immunization, and several other topics. It is the author's opinion that the Essentials Suite is the best overall PDA clinical reference tool for students and practicing clinicians.

The EBM side of Epocrates is the updated topics in the Dx portion and the CME feature where InfoPOEM and article summaries are downloaded frequently when the PDA is synced. The following screen shots will demonstrate how you would use Epocrates Essentials to help you diagnose and treat a 32-year-old female bank financial analyst who came to the emergency department with six hours of right-sided pleuritic chest pain and shortness of breath. A video demonstration of Epocrates Essentials, labeled Video 4–1, is available on the CD-ROM.

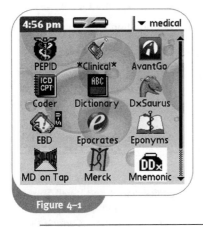

Figure 4–1

This is the Main Medical application screen with the icons grouped together.

Tap the stylized *e* for Epocrates to launch the program.

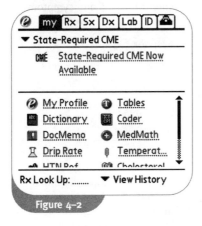

Figure 4–2

This screen shows the Epocrates Main menu tabs across the top with the following choices:

my—your home page

Rx—the drug and CAM therapy database

Sx—the symptom analyzer differential diagnosis generator

Dx—the 5-Minute Clinical Consult integrated with Rx and Sx

Lab—a lab test reference book with differentials linked to Dx diseases

ID—an infectious disease reference listing the best treatments by body system or infection

Doctor's bag icon—the extra programs you have elected to have including ACLS/ PALS guidelines, formulas, CME/EBM article summaries, and specialty programs

Tap on the Sx tab to enter the signs and symptoms analyzer.

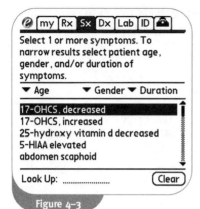

Figure 4-3

This is the Sx entry screen.

Tap Age and tap the 18–40 range.

Tap Gender and tap Female.

Tap Duration and tap the < 6-hour option

Tap the Look Up entry box and use the key pad to enter pleuritic.

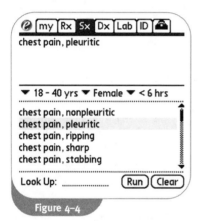

Figure 4-4

Chest pain, pleuritic is the best choice. Tap it and it will appear on the list above the age, gender, and duration. Continue to enter the signs and symptoms in the Look Up: box:

dyspnea

oral contraceptive ingestion

tachycardia

tachypnea

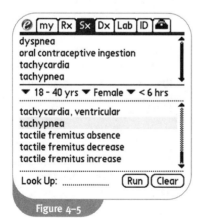

Figure 4-5

All the signs and symptoms listed in Figure 4–4 are now in the selected list above the age, gender, and duration.

Now click Run to analyze the symptoms together to formulate the most likely diagnosis.

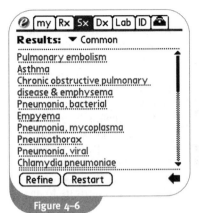

Figure 4-6

A differential diagnosis list of most common entities is generated as shown here. This list is hyperlinked to the full text of the Dx (5-Minute Consult).

Tap the Results: Common drop-down box toward the top of the screen and tap on Rare once it appears.

You can return to your existing list to add or subtract items by tapping the back arrow at the bottom left of the screen. If you tap Restart, you will erase your list and start over with no selections.

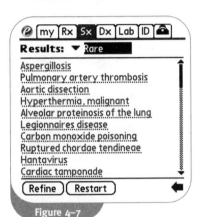

Figure 4-7

Shown in this screen are the rare causes of symptoms, and they are worth reviewing. All are linked to Dx by tapping a diagnosis.

Tap the Refine button at the bottom of the screen and a checklist of signs and symptoms will be presented that may help narrow the differential diagnosis.

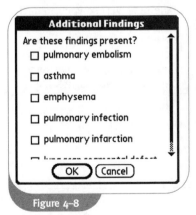

Figure 4-8

After reviewing the additional questions, you do not yet know about any positive responses, so return to your main list by tapping Cancel; then tap Common.

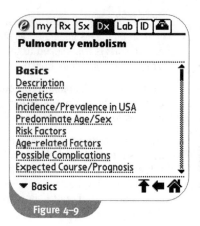
Figure 4-9

As seen in Figure 4–6, the most likely diagnosis and the most serious is pulmonary embolism. To find out the best workup, tap on Pulmonary embolism and see what is in the Dx or 5-Minute Clinical Consult. This is the opening screen for the Dx section on Pulmonay embolism. The Basics screen presents a submenu list that allows you to navigate to any part listed.

You may refresh your knowledge about the basics or navigate to the other subheadings by tapping the down arrow in the bottom right corner next to the word Basics.

The back arrow would take you to the differential diagnosis list in Sx, and tapping the house will take you to the Dx subject index.

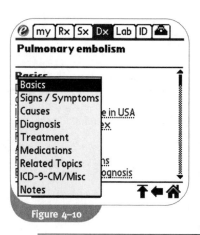
Figure 4-10

Each topic in Dx is arranged the same way so you can navigate to the information you want quickly. To answer the question about the best diagnostic workup for Pulmonary embolism, tap Diagnosis.

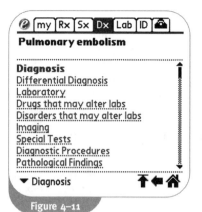

Figure 4-11

This subchapter structure is present in all topics. The Laboratory, Imaging, and Special Tests sections are the ones to tap next.

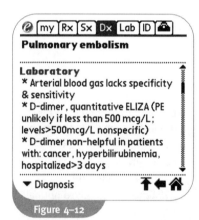

Figure 4-12

Use the scroll bar on the right side of the screen to read the text. You will see that a chest x-ray will help rule out other options in your differential diagnosis, such as pneumonia and pneumothorax. You order D-dimer ELIZA and imaging with either a V/Q lung scan or a spiral CT scan depending on what is available in your ED. You also order an EKG.

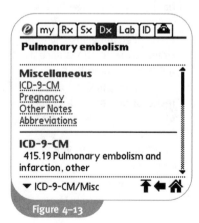

Figure 4-13

To get the ICD-9 code to put on the lab and radiology request, tap the drop-down box in the left lower corner and tap ICD-9-CM/Misc. The correct ICD-9 code is 415.19, the code needed in order for the lab or radiology to be reimbursed for the tests ordered.

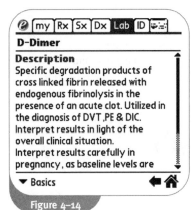

**Figure 4-14**

The D-Dimer test results come back while your patient is having a V/Q scan. The CXR and EKG were both normal. The D-Dimer value is greater than 0.5mcg/ml. You want to know all the causes so you tap on the Lab tab and enter D-d choosing D-Dimer. This screen is the test description.

Tap the drop-down arrow box in the lower left corner next to Basics to see the lab menu for any test.

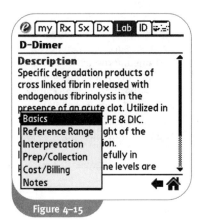

**Figure 4-15**

This is the lab menu that will pop up after tapping on the drop-down menu. It shows the sections you can navigate to:

Basics gives the test description and background.

Reference Range gives normal values.

Interpretation lists the differential diagnosis of high or low values.

Prep/Collection gives any lab collection instructions such as the type of blood tube.

Cost/Billing offers the average test cost and the ICD-9 codes of the disease you may be interested in.

Notes allows you to add your own input.

Now tap Interpretation.

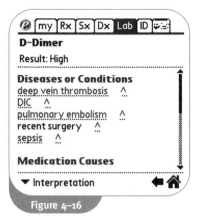

**Figure 4-16**

The Interpretation screen will list the diseases that cause an increased D-Dimer. The underlined diagnoses have a hyperlink to Dx if you want to read more details. Tapping the up arrow by each diagnosis will open a dialogue box with information on other tests to consider. The underlined tests are hyperlinked in the lab program if you want to read more.

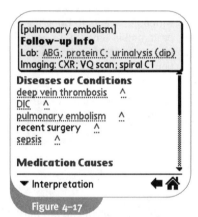

**Figure 4-17**

This text box is obtained by tapping the up arrow to the right of pulmonary embolism.

Tap on pulmonary embolism to go back to Dx to see what treatment is best.

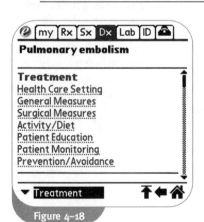

**Figure 4-18**

As depicted on this screen, the treatment section is divided into the same subcategories that helped you construct your patient orders as you admit your patient.

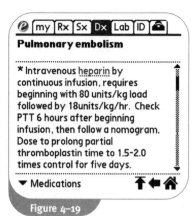

**Figure 4-19**

Tapping on the medication subsection within the menu options seen in Figure 4-10 brings up this screen, which provides specific pharmacologic treatments. Underlined medications are hyperlinked to the Rx section for more details and a drug-drug interaction calculator.

You choose to administer heparin by pump, monitoring her partial thromboplastin time (PTT) along with oral warfarin starting at 5 mg every day with adjustments to bring the prothrombin time INR to between two to three. Your patient should take the warfarin for 6 months.

Tap on the underlined heparin to go to Rx.

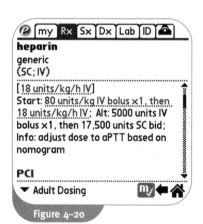

**Figure 4-20**

The Rx will show the adult dosing, and when you tap the underlined dose, a dosage calculator will appear to allow you to compute the dose based on the patient's weight and dosing schedule.

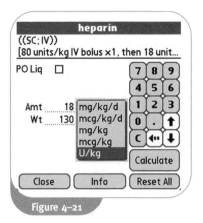

Figure 4-21

Tap on the Units box next to the Amt (Amount) line and you can choose mg/kg or, in this case, U/kg as highlighted.

Enter 18 in the Amount box (shown).

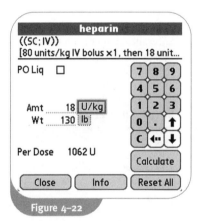

Figure 4-22

You can enter the patient's weight in kg or lb and change the units by tapping the lb or kg box. This saves another conversion calculation.

Tap Calculate and the results show 1062 U of heparin per hour for the pump setting.

Tap Close to go back into the Rx reference.

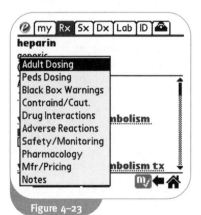

Figure 4-23

Tap the drop-down arrow in the bottom left of the screen (now hidden behind the menu box) and a standard menu common to all medications will appear. Review the adverse reactions to watch for by tapping on those words.

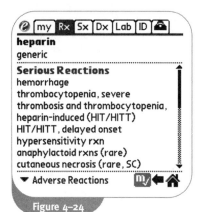

Figure 4-24

You quickly scan the list presented and are reminded about heparin-induced thrombocytopenia (HIT); you will monitor her platelet count daily along with her PTT and PT.

Next, tap the M checkbox for doing a drug interaction calculation.

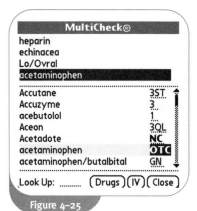

Figure 4-25

Enter all the medications the patient is taking by entering the first few letters and choosing the drug from the list. When all are listed, tap the Drugs button at the bottom of the screen to start the cross check.

The IV button will list intravenous incompatibilities.

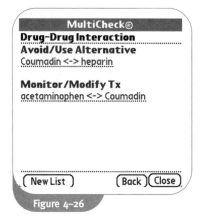

Figure 4-26

You knew about the additive anticoagulation effects of Coumadin and heparin. You tap on the underlined interaction to see an information box warning you to watch the acetaminophen dosing because of increased INR from the hepatic metabolism.

You know now that the echinacea is not an issue.

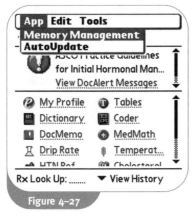

Figure 4-27

Other features from the My Home Page screen include setting your memory management and storing part of the program on a memory card (recommended).

AutoUpdate allows you to get the latest updates without doing a PC-PDA sync if you have a wireless or cell-connected PDA.

The Tools tab allows you set your preferences for your screen selection and defaults.

## PEPID

PEPID is an integrated program developed by emergency medicine physicians to meet their needs for quick, evidence-based information. There are multiple PEPID versions including Emergency Physician Suite, Primary Care Plus (PCP), Clinical Rotation Companion, Pediatrics Module, and several nursing products. The PCP product is the closest comparison to Epocrates Essentials. There are 2300 disease and trauma topics with diagnosis, pathophysiology, treatment, and disposition written by PEPID authors. Protocols for emergency life-saving procedures, quick drugs and drips, toxidromes, and algorithms all are included and grouped in the emergency section. The program also includes 400 evidence-based medicine topics from clinical inquiries and help-desk answers with over 600 integrated recommendations.

A toxicology section covers toxin identification: drugs of abuse; household and cleaning agents; plants, mushrooms, and seafood; pests, rodent, and herbicides; inhaled gases; heavy metals and caustics; medication overdoses, and antidotes.

In addition, there is weapons of mass destruction diagnostic and treatment information on the nuclear, chemical, and biological weapon threats primary care providers may encounter.

PEPID includes 200 anatomical illustrations and rhythm strips for teaching patients or students.

The drug database includes over 6000 drug, herbal, and over-the-counter (OTC) generic and trade names with extensive kinetics and mechanism-of-action information, adult and pediatric dosing with built-in dosing calculators (weight-based, body surface area-based, even IV-drip rate calculators), overdose management, and trade/cost information. Users can cross reference up to 40 drugs, herbal remedies, and OTC medications simultaneously in the drug interactions module. A medical calculator index contains 3000 formulas.

PEPID Online, Wireless, and Wireless Mobile content is continuously updated without downloads. PEPID releases free content updates and application upgrades to PDA software subscribers on a regular basis (approximately every 8–10 weeks). Subscribers can view and download the most current update on their "My Account" page simply by logging in at www.pepid.com.

Using the earlier patient case, a 32-year-old female presents to the emergency room with 6 hours of right-sided pleuritic chest pain and shortness of breath. We will answer the same questions using the PEPID–PCP. A video demonstration of PEPID, labeled Video 4–2, is available on the CD-ROM.

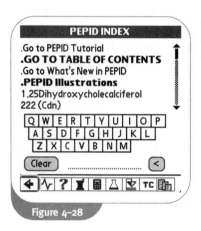

Figure 4-28

PEPID opens with an index and a screen tap keyboard to enter search terms.

Along the bottom are quick links:

The back arrow returns you to the previous screen.

The EKG symbol provides emergency guides.

The ? icon lists information on how to use PEPID, and provides a quick reference plus abbreviations and illustrations.

The mortar icon denotes the drug interaction generator.

The calculator symbol offers medical calculations.

A tap on the chemistry flask leads you to the lab reference, an extra purchase.

The down arrow provides a quick link menu.

The TC tab denotes the table of contents.

The paper notes provides a place to add your own notes.

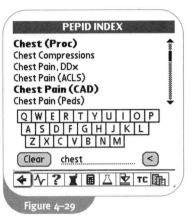

Figure 4-29

If you type in pleuritic for the differential diagnosis, you will not find it because it is not present in the search index.

However, type in the phrase chest pain without the descriptor pleuritic and you will see the list of choices as shown on the screen.

Chest Pain DDx
Chest Pain (ACLS)
Chest Pain (CAD)
Chest Pain (Peds)

Next, tap on Chest Pain, DDx to see the differential diagnosis.

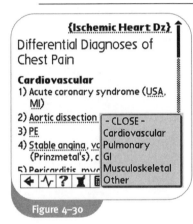

Figure 4-30

All the causes of chest pain organized by body system are listed. This screen shows the cardiovascular causes. All the underlined diseases are hyper-linked to text references.

Tap on PE (Pulmonary Embo-lus) because that is what you suspect.

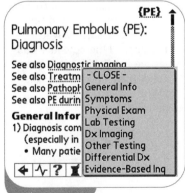

Figure 4-31

PEPID disease text has the same menu structure for every disease.

The submenu appears automatically.

Tap on Lab Testing and Dx Imaging to see the workup.

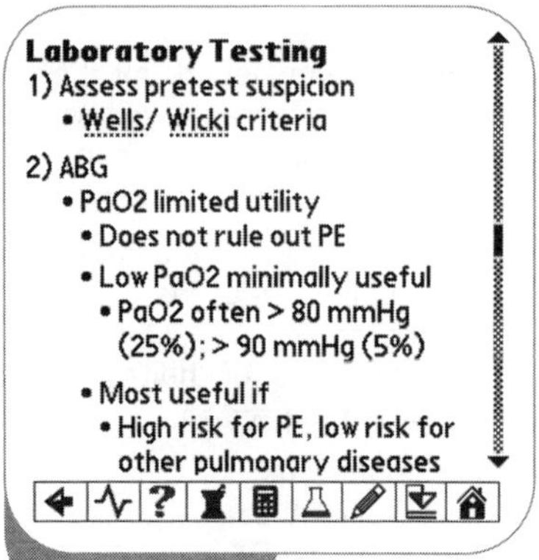

**Laboratory Testing**
1) Assess pretest suspicion
   • Wells/ Wicki criteria
2) ABG
   • PaO2 limited utility
   • Does not rule out PE
   • Low PaO2 minimally useful
     • PaO2 often > 80 mmHg
       (25%); > 90 mmHg (5%)
   • Most useful if
     • High risk for PE, low risk for
       other pulmonary diseases

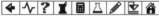

Figure 4-32

When you tap on the words Laboratory Testing, a comprehensive list of diagnostic tests with evidence-based recommendations comes on the screen. There are links for Wells/Wicki criteria, which is an evidence-based diagnosis algorithm for the likely probability of having a PE if there are certain findings.

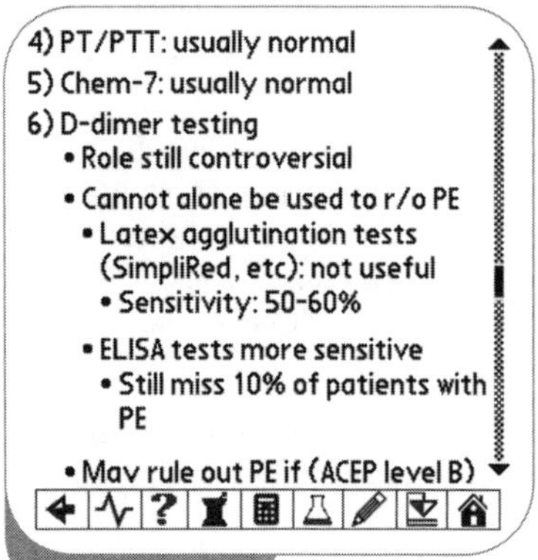

---

4) PT/PTT: usually normal
5) Chem-7: usually normal
6) D-dimer testing
   • Role still controversial
   • Cannot alone be used to r/o PE
     • Latex agglutination tests
       (SimpliRed, etc): not useful
     • Sensitivity: 50-60%
   • ELISA tests more sensitive
     • Still miss 10% of patients with
       PE
   • May rule out PE if (ACEP level B)

Figure 4-33

Moving the scroll arrow downward reveals more test options including the evidence.

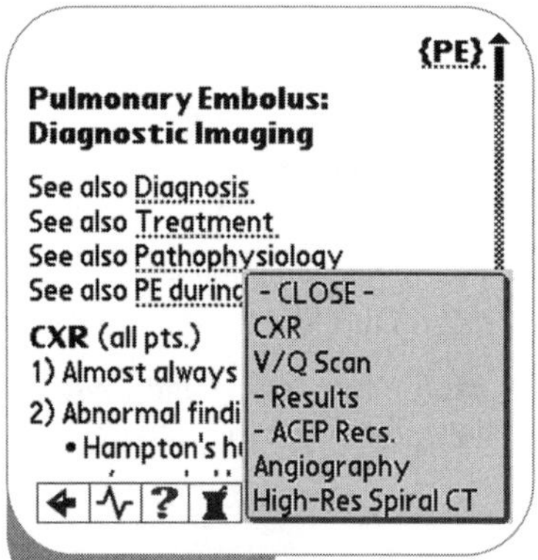

---

{PE}

**Pulmonary Embolus:
Diagnostic Imaging**

See also Diagnosis
See also Treatment
See also Pathophysiology
See also PE during   - CLOSE -
                       CXR
CXR (all pts.)         V/Q Scan
1) Almost always       - Results
2) Abnormal findi      - ACEP Recs.
   • Hampton's h        Angiography
                       High-Res Spiral CT

Figure 4-34

From the main menu in Figure 4–31, tap Dx Imaging to see this screen. Under Diagnostic Imaging, all the potential studies are listed with the pros and cons. The menu box appears in the lower right screen automatically.

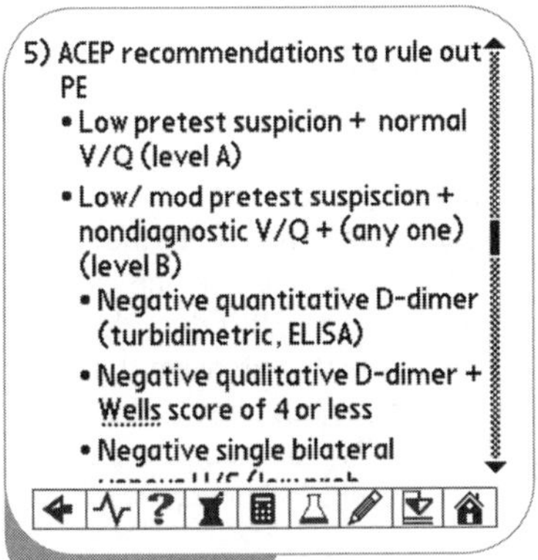

5) ACEP recommendations to rule out
   PE
   • Low pretest suspicion + normal
     V/Q (level A)
   • Low/ mod pretest suspiscion +
     nondiagnostic V/Q + (any one)
     (level B)
     • Negative quantitative D-dimer
       (turbidimetric, ELISA)
     • Negative qualitative D-dimer +
       Wells score of 4 or less
   • Negative single bilateral

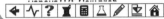

Figure 4-35

As shown on this screen, the American College of Emergency Physicians (ACEP) evidence-based recommendations are listed with the level of evidence. PEPID has its origins in emergency medicine and has a very comprehensive database for emergency problems.

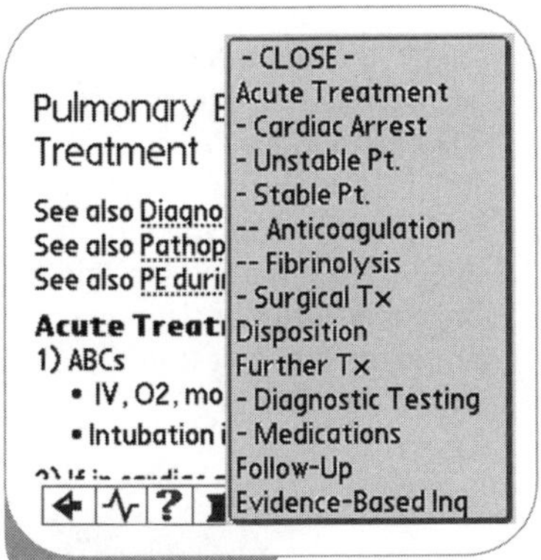

---

Pulmonary E
Treatment

See also Diagno
See also Pathop
See also PE durii

**Acute Treatı**
1) ABCs
   • IV, O2, mo
   • Intubation i

- CLOSE -
Acute Treatment
- Cardiac Arrest
- Unstable Pt.
- Stable Pt.
-- Anticoagulation
-- Fibrinolysis
- Surgical Tx
Disposition
Further Tx
- Diagnostic Testing
- Medications
Follow-Up
Evidence-Based Inq

Figure 4-36

An automatic treatment menu appears, which allows navigation to the most applicable area.

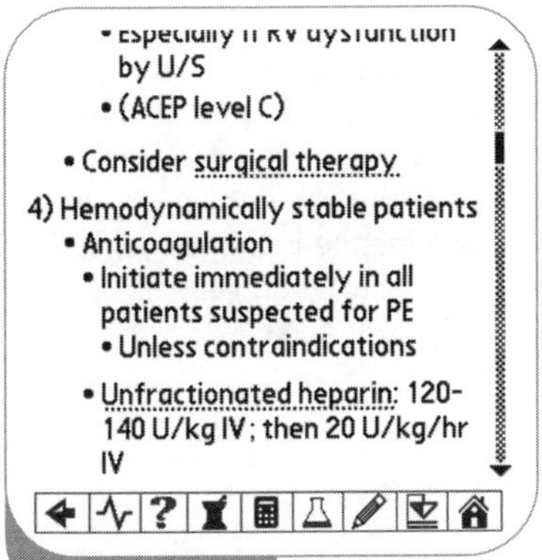

---

• Especially if RV dysfunction
  by U/S
• (ACEP level C)

• Consider surgical therapy

4) Hemodynamically stable patients
   • Anticoagulation
     • Initiate immediately in all
       patients suspected for PE
     • Unless contraindications

   • Unfractionated heparin: 120-
     140 U/kg IV; then 20 U/kg/hr
     IV

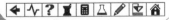

Figure 4-37

Scrolling down through the treatment options for hemodynamically stable patients, we see Unfractionated heparin. Tapping on heparin or any underlined medication leads you to detailed drug information.

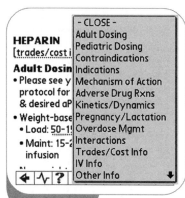

Figure 4-38

Tapping on Unfractionated heparin in Figure 4–37 brings you to this screen, which shows the drug details and the automatic submenu within the drug information section. The content for the PEPID drug database is more extensive than Epocrates, but it lacks the formulary lists or Medicare part D list present in Epocrates.

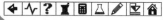

Figure 4-39

This is the Adult Dosing screen. Any underlined dose will link to a dose calculator. This built-in dosing calculator is activated when you tap the underlined dose and the drip calculator for IV dosing, displayed as drops next to the phrase IV infusion.

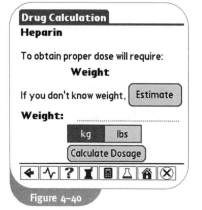

Figure 4-40

The calculator stores the dosing of the drug you are looking at, so all you need to do is enter the patient's weight. A nice feature is the weight estimator based on gender, height, and age.

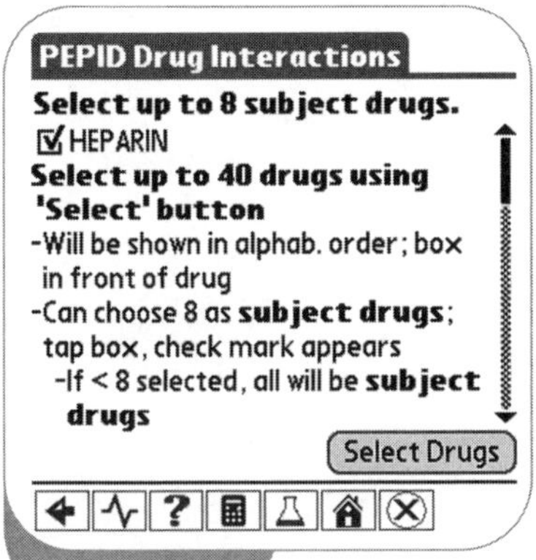

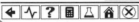

**PEPID Drug Interactions**

**Select up to 8 subject drugs.**
☑ HEPARIN
**Select up to 40 drugs using**
**'Select' button**
-Will be shown in alphab. order; box
 in front of drug
-Can choose 8 as **subject drugs**;
 tap box, check mark appears
 -If < 8 selected, all will be **subject**
  **drugs**

[ Select Drugs ]

Figure 4-41

A drug interaction calculator allows you to select eight drugs from a listing. Tap on the drugs you wish to add to the list and tap Done when all drugs have been selected.

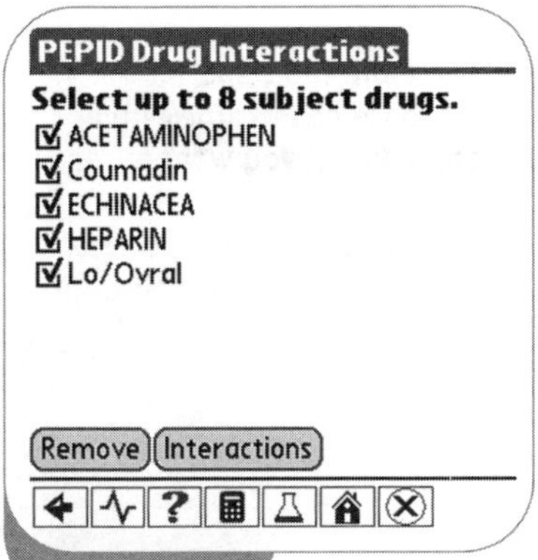

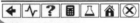

**PEPID Drug Interactions**

**Select up to 8 subject drugs.**
☑ ACETAMINOPHEN
☑ Coumadin
☑ ECHINACEA
☑ HEPARIN
☑ Lo/Ovral

[ Remove ] [ Interactions ]

Figure 4-42

Your list will be displayed (an example is shown here) and the program will look for interactions for the up to eight checked drugs. You can have a longer list, but you can only select a maximum of eight at a time. Tap Interactions to run the program.

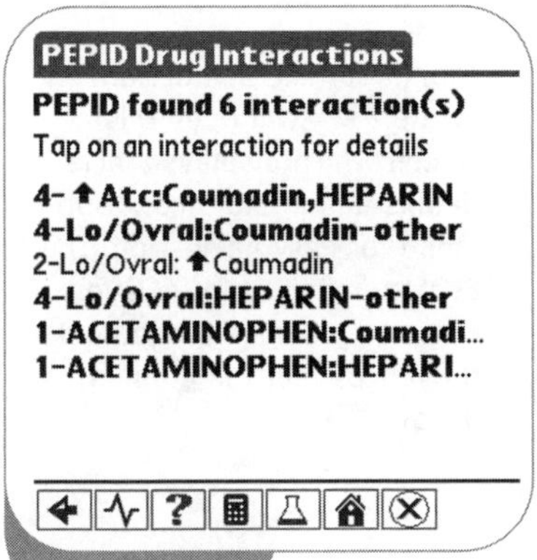

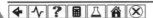

**PEPID Drug Interactions**

**PEPID found 6 interaction(s)**
Tap on an interaction for details

**4- ↑Atc:Coumadin,HEPARIN**
**4-Lo/Ovral:Coumadin-other**
2-Lo/Ovral: ↑Coumadin
**4-Lo/Ovral:HEPARIN-other**
**1-ACETAMINOPHEN:Coumadi...**
**1-ACETAMINOPHEN:HEPARI...**

Figure 4-43

This screen shows the results in order of importance, where 4 is a significant interaction and 1 is an insignificant one. Tap on the interactions to see additional details.

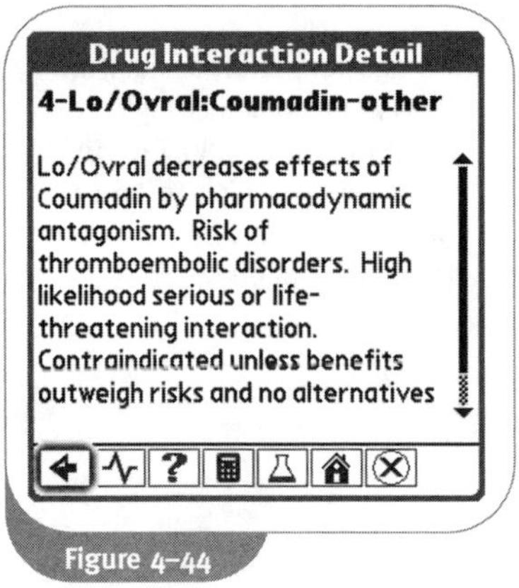

**Drug Interaction Detail**

**4-Lo/Ovral:Coumadin-other**

Lo/Ovral decreases effects of Coumadin by pharmacodynamic antagonism. Risk of thromboembolic disorders. High likelihood serious or life-threatening interaction. Contraindicated unless benefits outweigh risks and no alternatives

Figure 4–44

This is the Drug Interaction Detail screen.

---

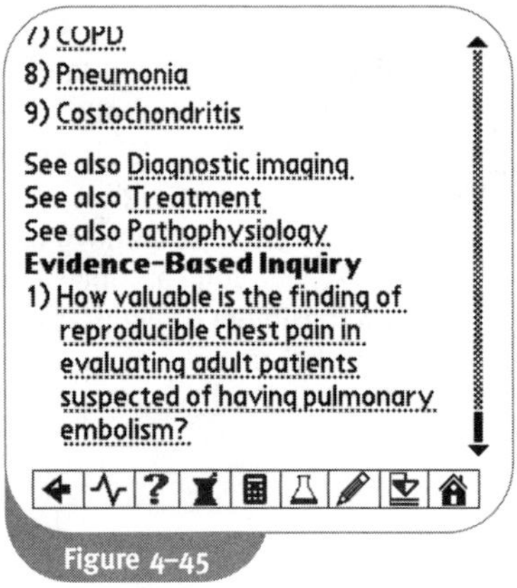

7) COPD
8) Pneumonia
9) Costochondritis

See also Diagnostic imaging
See also Treatment
See also Pathophysiology
**Evidence-Based Inquiry**
1) How valuable is the finding of reproducible chest pain in evaluating adult patients suspected of having pulmonary embolism?

Figure 4–45

There are topic-specific evidence-based articles that are linked if you want to read them. This is an excellent feature not present in Epocrates. See the example as shown in this figure.

---

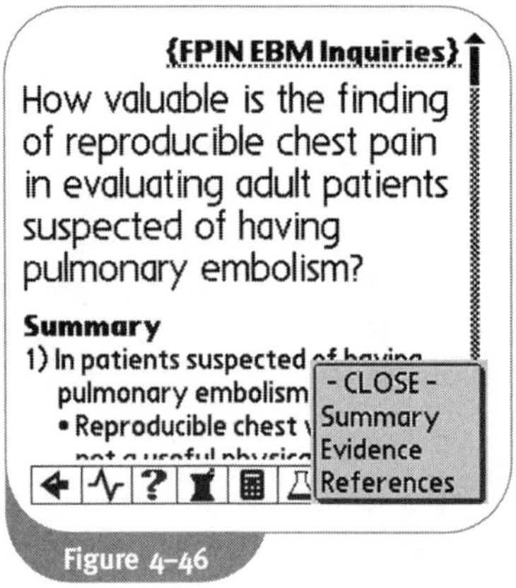

**{FPIN EBM Inquiries}**

How valuable is the finding of reproducible chest pain in evaluating adult patients suspected of having pulmonary embolism?

**Summary**
1) In patients suspected of having
pulmonary embolism
  • Reproducible chest

- CLOSE -
Summary
Evidence
References

Figure 4–46

Tapping article number one in Figure 4–45 will open this screen which displays article details and an automatic sub-menu for easy navigation. The EBM summary is in PICO format and provides the journal references that the authors used.

---

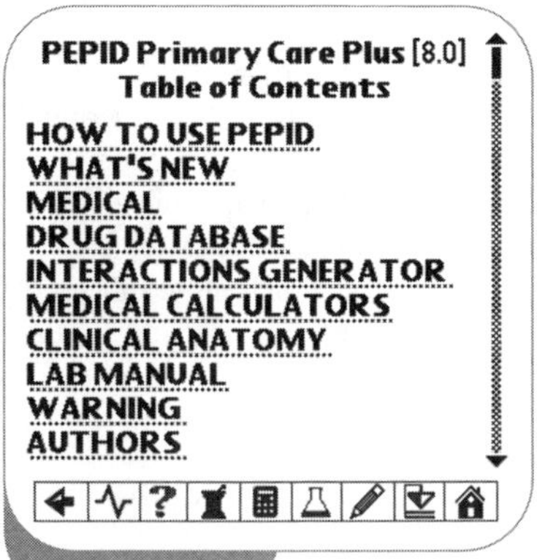

**PEPID Primary Care Plus [8.0]**
**Table of Contents**

HOW TO USE PEPID
WHAT'S NEW
MEDICAL
DRUG DATABASE
INTERACTIONS GENERATOR
MEDICAL CALCULATORS
CLINICAL ANATOMY
LAB MANUAL
WARNING
AUTHORS

Figure 4-47

To get to the ICD-9 codes for PE, tap on the house at the bottom of the screen to go to the main menu. Once there, tap on MEDICAL (in the list as shown).

---

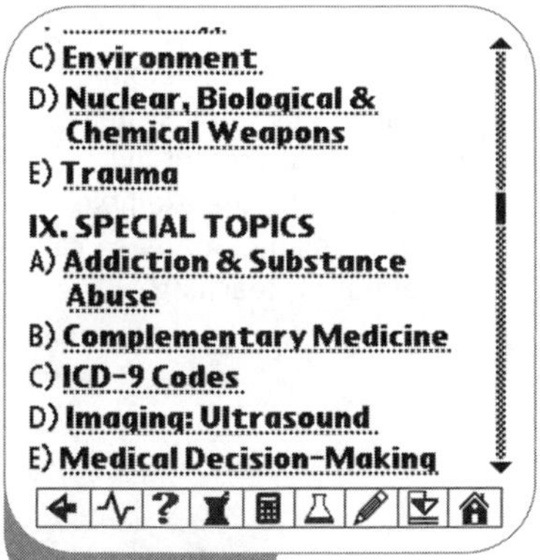

C) **Environment**
D) **Nuclear, Biological &**
   **Chemical Weapons**
E) **Trauma**

**IX. SPECIAL TOPICS**
A) **Addiction & Substance**
   **Abuse**
B) **Complementary Medicine**
C) **ICD-9 Codes**
D) **Imaging: Ultrasound**
E) **Medical Decision-Making**

Figure 4-48

Within the Medical submenus, there is an ICD-9 codes listing. Tap on this underlined feature to see a listing of body systems from which to make your selection.

---

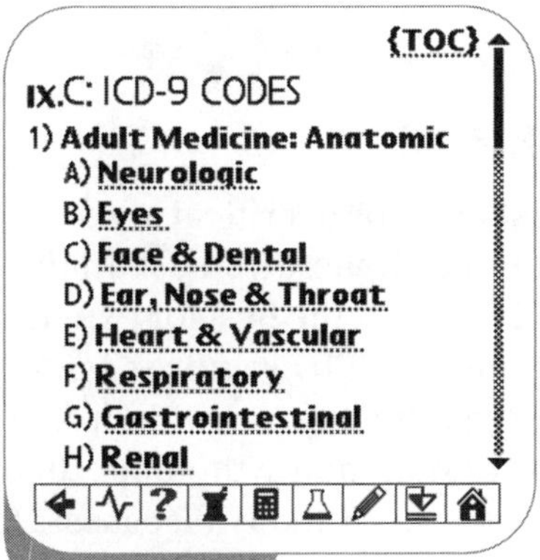

{TOC}

**IX.C: ICD-9 CODES**
1) **Adult Medicine: Anatomic**
   A) **Neurologic**
   B) **Eyes**
   C) **Face & Dental**
   D) **Ear, Nose & Throat**
   E) **Heart & Vascular**
   F) **Respiratory**
   G) **Gastrointestinal**
   H) **Renal**

Figure 4-49

The proper body system is Respiratory to get to the pulmonary embolus ICD-9 code.

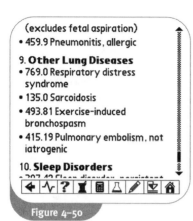

(excludes fetal aspiration)
- 459.9 Pneumonitis, allergic

9. **Other Lung Diseases**
- 769.0 Respiratory distress syndrome
- 135.0 Sarcoidosis
- 493.81 Exercise-induced bronchospasm
- 415.19 Pulmonary embolism, not iatrogenic

10. **Sleep Disorders**

Figure 4–50

Finally, you arrive at the PE ICD-9 code under Other. Many find having the ICD-9 code listed within each disease description as in Epocrates DX and Lab is much more efficient for lookups.

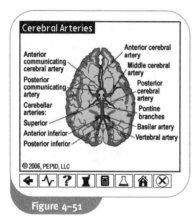

Figure 4–51

PEPID has several anatomic illustrations by body system and EKGs that are not in Epocrates. Like the example shown in this figure, these can be helpful for teaching.

## Summary of Integrated Programs

Both of these programs allow for fast lookups of critical and useful information. It is the author's opinion that Epocrates Essentials is the most well rounded for everyone and PEPID is the best for experienced emergency or critical care practitioners. PEPID requires some basic knowledge of what you want, whereas Epocrates will help the user formulate a differential diagnosis from signs and symptoms, then lead the user to more information about the most likely diseases. One or both of these products should be the foundation EBM reference in your PDA library.

# The Internet-
# EBM-PDA Web
# Sites

# 5

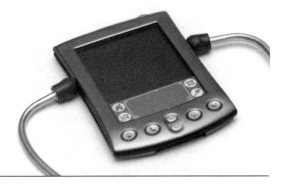

## Objectives

■ Explore Web resources available for a Web-enabled cell phone or wireless PDA.

■ Learn how to use the tools that allow Web site contents to be "clipped" and stored on a PDA for reference.

■ Learn how to effectively search Medline, a vast resource for all of the world's medical journal articles.

■ Learn how to navigate EBM Web sites designed for the PC with a Web-enabled PDA.

## Internet Resources for the Web-Enabled PDA

The Internet has revolutionized medical knowledge with an explosion of resources for practicing clinicians and patients. The Internet is the fastest way to update medical knowledge. There is a multitude of free and credible EBM resources the busy clinician can access using his or her PDA at the bedside or the clinic.

## Internet Browsers and Web Clipping

There are many excellent free Web sites that provide evidence-based information through Web-connected PDAs. Wireless Web or cell phone access may not be available in each setting where medical care is delivered, so these sites may be of limited use. Downloading Web pages to a PDA allows you to read the Web content later when you are not connected. This a great tool for getting the latest medical journal abstracts to your Palm or Windows PDA or clipping Web books that are viewable using PC-Web browsers.

■ Using AvantGo Web Clipping

AvantGo, at www.AvantGo.com, is a free Web-clipping service that downloads Web pages to your PDA when you sync to a Web-connected PC or wirelessly using cell phone services or a wireless Web access.

You will need to do a brief registration to set up a user name and password. You may download the PDA software on your PC and install it on your PDA at your next sync. Using your Web-connected PC, you can subscribe to channels that provide news, weather, sports, computer news, and medical news. You can search the channels, which are PDA-friendly Web sites, using the key word "medical," and you will see timely topics on medicine and American medical news, as well as medical journal abstracts from Wiley Interscience Mobile Edition.

If you know the URLs (the "www" address) of Web sites that have excellent content, you can make that Web site one of your channels. Using your Web-connected PC, log in at AvantGo and click on the "Create Personal Channel" option. There, you will complete a Web form with the name of the Web site, the Web site URL, the maximum size of all the Web page text and images up to the limit of 2000K with a free account, and the link depth you wish to download (how many levels of pages linked below the main menu page for the program to download). You can also designate whether you want the program to follow off-site links (it is best to say no if you do not want the program to copy links to other Web sites) and whether the program should include images (to which you would answer yes if you want to download all images). You want this to update at every sync if the material is continuously being updated, or you can enter an interval if it is fairly static. Finally, click on the Save Channel button.

A good example of the Web-clipping technique is to add the American College of Physicians (ACP) Medicine BestDx/Best Rx Web site at http://www.acpmedicine.com/dxrx/dxrxpromo1.htm. It is a free (at the time of this writing), point-of-care clinical recommendation that is evidence-based. The maximum size of the text downloaded to the PDA is 600K, and the link depth is set to one. Set off-site links to no if you do not want links to other Web sites copied.

The following screens will show you how to configure AvantGo on your PC and on a Palm PDA to copy the Web book *ACP Medicine RxDx*. Video demonstrations of AvantGo, labeled Video 5–1, and Video 5–2, are available on the CD-ROM.

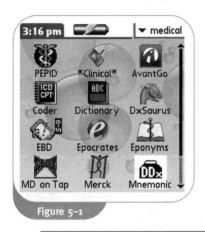

Install AvantGo after completing the free registration. You then select what Web content or channels you want downloaded to your PDA. The AvantGo icon looks like a highway (see the icon in the upper right corner of the screen).

Figure 5–1

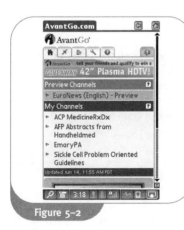

The channels you have selected will be displayed on the main menu (see the example shown).

As an example, the ACP MedicineRxDx were the Web pages selected as a channel on the AvantGo Web site when the sample person registered.

Figure 5–2

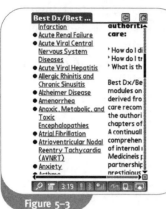

**Figure 5-3**

Shown here is the main menu for BestDx/BestRx.

Each underlined topic is linked to another Web page with the text content. Scrolling down the page and tapping on Acute Viral Hepatitis brings up that topic page.

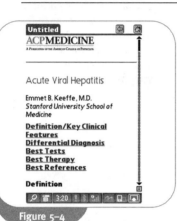

**Figure 5-4**

The topic page (shown here for Acute Viral Hepatitis) is a summary that has the sub-headings listed. This is typical of most topics. You can tap on any of the topic headings to go directly to that text.

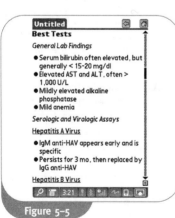

**Figure 5-5**

Tapping on the Best Tests section (as seen in Figure 5-4) will bring up a list of tests and expected results (a sample of those tests is shown).

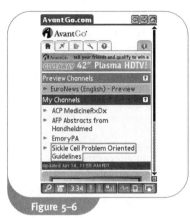

Figure 5–6

If you have the ability or knowledge to create Web sites, you can create your own Web book and make it an AvantGo channel. In this example, problem-oriented guidelines for sickle cell disease were posted to share this information with clinicians worldwide who treat sickle cell patients.

AvantGo allows the clinician to record the Web pages to their PDA and allows updates when the PDA is synced to a Web-connected PC. The Web pages can be updated any time and all the AvantGo PDA books will be updated automatically.

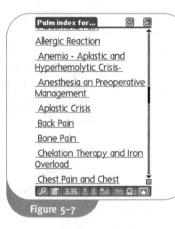

Figure 5–7

Design a PDA table of contents where each tile is linked to a text-based guideline (see the example shown). AvantGo keeps the links intact and copies all the linked pages to the PDA to the depth you specify (one page below, two pages below, etc.).

It is best not to include many pictures or complex columns when designing Web pages for PDAs because they take a long time to load and may fill the entire screen.

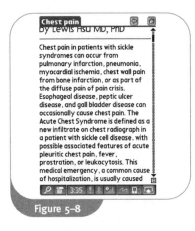

**Chest pain**

by Lewis Hsu MD, PhD

Chest pain in patients with sickle
syndromes can occur from
pulmonary infarction, pneumonia,
myocardial ischemia, chest wall pain
from bone infarction, or as part of
the diffuse pain of pain crisis.
Esophageal disease, peptic ulcer
disease, and gall bladder disease can
occasionally cause chest pain. The
Acute Chest Syndrome is defined as a
new infiltrate on chest radiograph in
a patient with sickle cell disease, with
possible associated features of acute
pleuritic chest pain, fever,
prostration, or leukocytosis. This
medical emergency, a common cause
of hospitalization, is usually caused

3:35

Figure 5-8

This is an example of the guideline format. This Web reference has been saved as a PDA e-book. Any time the Web page is updated, AvantGo will send the updated pages to the PDA.

This is an excellent way for teaching programs or hospitals to send updated schedules, notes, or information to student's or staff's PDAs by using one Web site to which they all have access.

## Web Browsing

Web connected computers have revolutionized the availability of medical knowledge. The Web-enabled PDA brings the resources of the Internet to the bedside where computers may not be available. Both wireless and cell phone–equipped Palm and Windows PDAs come with Web browsing software that allows you to view live Web pages on your PDA when you can be connected. Web pages with large pictures will load slowly and will be difficult to navigate on the small PDA screen. It is faster to choose the no picture–no graphics option if you do not need them. There are PDA-friendly Web pages that minimize the graphics and make the text easy to read and navigate.

## Web EBM Search Tools

There are PDA programs that can help you quickly search the Internet for evidence-based medical information. The search tools described here are free at the time of this writing.

■ National Library of Medicine: PubMed for Handhelds

The world's largest online collection of biomedical journal article abstracts and links to full text articles is available at the National Library of Medicine (NLM) at www.nlm.nih.gov/. It is the author's opinion that the easiest to use search tool for this massive database is PubMed. A free PDA program called MD on Tap for Palm or Windows can be downloaded at www.nlm.nih.gov/mobile/; to use the PDA Web browser, go to http://pubmedhh.nlm.nih.gov/nlm/ and bookmark this page for a PDA-friendly Web page.

You have a patient with recurrent angina and want to see the latest studies about using the platelet blocker clopidogrel compared to using aspirin. The following screen shots demonstrate the lookup using the PubMed Web site with a Palm PDA. A video demonstration of MD on Tap, labeled Video 5–3 is available on the CD-ROM.

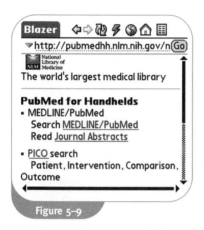

Figure 5–9

Shown here is the opening menu at PubMed for PDAs; you can do a search, read abstracts for journals you select, and even do a PICO-formatted EBM question.

Using your PDA Web browser in a wireless or cell-connected area allows live searches of Medline through PubMed, the simple search tool that inquires the Medline database.

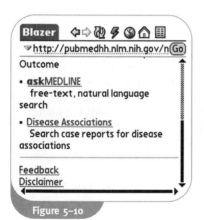

Figure 5–10

There is a free-text, natural language ("plain" English) search tool that provides results to simple questions. There also is a disease-association tool that will let you know if a sign or symptom is associated with a specific disease.

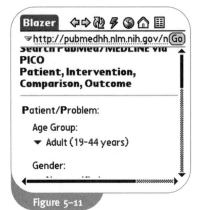

Figure 5-11

Doing a PICO-formatted question, select the age group from the drop-down menu. Then enter the gender.

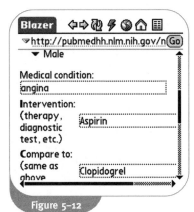

Figure 5-12

Enter the medical condition you are interested in, such as angina, and the interventions you want to compare, such as aspirin and clopidogrel preventive therapy.

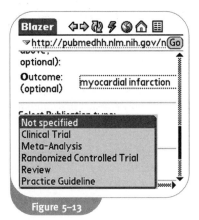

Figure 5-13

The outcome you want to happen or prevent with your intervention is the last input. In this example, you want to prevent myocardial infarction. The type of articles you want to have in the search is presented in an automatic pop-up menu. As shown in this choice, you chose "Not specified" to give the maximum results.

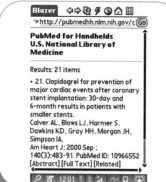

Figure 5-14

This search strategy provided 21 articles for review. Scroll through the titles and tap on the abstract tab (in this example, located at the bottom of the screen) to be linked to the article abstract text.

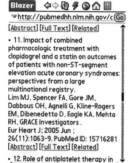

Figure 5-15

Here is a more recent article published in 2005.

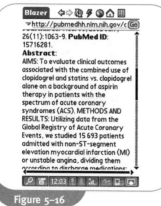

Figure 5-16

Shown here is the abstract text for the 2005 article that summarizes the results.

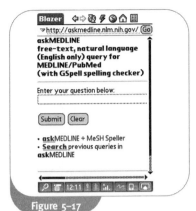

Figure 5-17

Another search method is available using "plain" English. This program will check your spelling and offer suggestions to increase the accuracy of your results.

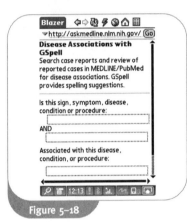

Figure 5-18

Another tool available will allow you to inquire about signs, symptoms, and lab results with certain disease states or procedures.

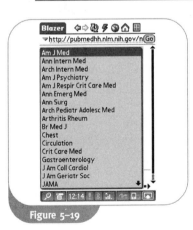

Figure 5-19

Tapping the read journal abstracts option on the PubMed home page (Figure 5–9) allows you to select a journal from a drop-down menu. A sample listing is shown here.

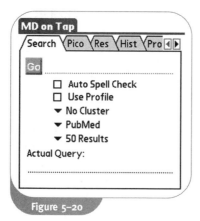

Figure 5-20

If you do not have continuous wireless access to PubMed, MD on Tap is a free program from the National Library of Medicine that you can download to your PDA. This requires a Web connection, but you can construct your query offline and do the search when you have Web access. After tapping the MD on Tap icon on the PDA program menu, you will see this opening screen. It shows that this program has many of the same options as the Web version of PubMed.

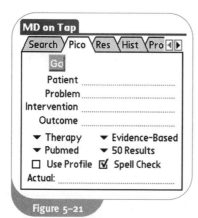

Figure 5-21

This screen shows the PICO-formatted menu for the user to fill in the blanks. There are some drop-down submenus on which to tap in your answers.

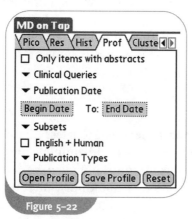

Figure 5-22

Preferences can be set in the Prof (Profile) section that will limit the search and exclude criteria you set.

■ WISER: Wireless Information System for Emergency Responders

Wireless Information System for Emergency Responders (WISER) is a free PDA program from the National Library of Medicine designed to assist first responders in hazardous material incidents. WISER provides a wide range of information on hazardous substances, including substance identification support, physical characteristics, human health information, and containment and suppression advice. It can be found at http://wiser.nlm.nih.gov/. There is a Web version for use when connected and a freestanding program version you can download to your PDA for use offline. This is a valuable resource for providers in the emergency department or EMS.

■ AIDSinfo's PDA Tools

If you have patients on HIV therapy, there is a free tool sponsored by AIDSinfo to prevent drug toxicity and capture the latest treatment protocols. The site (http://aidsinfo.nih.gov/PDATools/Default.aspx?MenuItem=AIDSinfoTools) includes the Antiretroviral Toxicity Tool for Pocket PCs and federally approved medical guidelines for PDAs. The documents are in PDF format, so you will need the free Adobe Reader for your PDA. Download it from Adobe at www.adobe.com/products/reader/.

■ Clinical Trials

This is a Web-based search page that will allow you to enter a medical condition and see all the clinical trials in progress. The details of the trials have clinical summaries for the rationale and references. This is an excellent way to see who, where, and what is on the cutting edge. You also might refer your patient to this site for the latest research.

**How to find the best place to refer your patient for the latest clinical trial.** You have a patient who has just been diagnosed with multiple myeloma and he would like to have the latest treatments done in a center near his home in Atlanta, Georgia. You have a bookmark in your PDA browser for http://clinicaltrials.gov/. At that site, you would see the following.

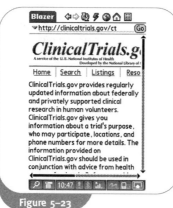
Figure 5-23

Shown here is the home page for ClinicalTrials.gov.

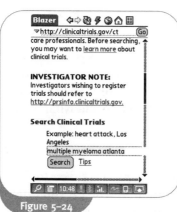
Figure 5-24

Scroll down to the search box at the bottom of the page. Enter the disease you want to learn about. In addition, you may list your nearest city to help in locating the closest clinical trial.

In this example, you would enter multiple myeloma and Atlanta to find the resources for your patient.

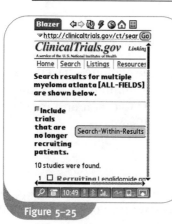
Figure 5-25

Ten studies were found in this search. Scroll though the list to see who, what, and where the trials cover and are located. The status of the study will be listed so you know who is doing the recruiting.

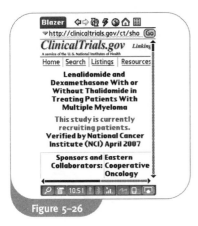

Shown on this screen is one of the studies currently recruiting patients in the Atlanta area.

**Figure 5-26**

### ■ Free Medical Textbooks

There are multiple full-text Web books covering several medical topics available on the NLM Web site at www.ncbi.nlm.nih.gov/entrez/query.fcgi?db=books that can be viewed with your Web browser. The list of available books is expanding, so visit often to see what is available.

### ■ Google

PDA Google at www.google.com/pda is a great search tool that will identify many Web sources of information. However, you must check the sources and weed through the sites that do not help and that are not from credible sources.

## PDA-Friendly Medical Web Sites for Clinicians

The following Web sites are excellent, free evidence-based resources that are accessible with a PC or a Web-enabled PDA. Some of the screens are not optimized for a small PDA screen and may require horizontal and vertical scrolling to see all content.

### ■ EMedicine

EMedicine at www.emedicine.com is a free-access online open-source Web textbook with 10,000 contributors writing over 6500 articles in all areas of medicine. Operated by WebMD, it is continually updated. A search tool or a browse-by-specialty option is available to find the topic of interest. Each topic is divided into the following sections:

Authors and editors

Introduction

Clinical

Differentials

Workup

Treatment

Medication

Follow-up

Miscellaneous

Multimedia

References

You have a patient you suspect has pancreatitis and you want to do a quick review using eMedicine. These are the screen shots you would see on a Palm PDA.

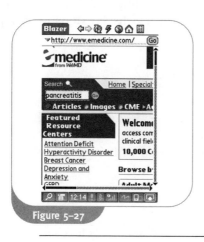

Figure 5–27

This is the home page for eMedicine. The search box is where you enter the topic you want information about; as shown for this example, pancreatitis. Next, tap the Go button next to the search box.

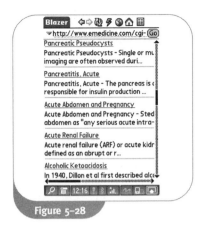

EMedicine is designed to be an e-book with chapters. A list of chapters related to the search term is displayed in this screen.

Tap on Pancreatitis, Acute and you will be linked to a full text chapter.

Figure 5-28

A differential diagnosis tool is located at www.emedicine.com/diagnosis.shtml. There are extensive, free continuing medical education activities for clinicians who register. However, most of these are better to do on a Web-connected PC.

■ MedicalStudent.com

MedicalStudent.com at www.medicalstudent.com/ is a Web site with a rich collection of Web resources, free online textbooks, medical dictionaries, and programs that benefit students and practicing clinicians. It is worth browsing the links and bookmarking Web textbooks that might be useful in your studies. Use your PDA browser to view the Web link on your Web-connected PDA. The list is extensive, grouped by specialty, and is updated periodically.

■ UConn Health Center Medical Library Links

The University of Connecticut Health Center Medical Library offers PDA links at their Web site, http://library.uchc.edu/pda. This is an extensive list of PDA resources with Palm/Windows designations to indicate from which platform the program will work. The Web links are grouped by medical specialty and topics.

■ The Cochrane Collaboration

The Cochrane Collection at www.cochrane.org is a well-respected peer-reviewed, regularly updated collection of evidence-based medicine databases, including the Cochrane Database of Systematic Reviews. Summaries are available for free.

■ American College of Physicians Journal Club

The general purpose of the American College of Physicians (ACP) Journal Club, at www.acpjc.org, is to select from over 100 journals the articles that report original studies and systematic reviews relevant for clinicians in internal medicine. These articles are summarized in value-added abstracts and commented on by clinical experts. The Web site has the full text of the paper edition for Web-enabled PDAs. You will need to pay a subscription fee to obtain a login and password to access the materials.

The ACP also produces a PDA-EBM reference called PIER that is distributed by STAT!Ref. It will be discussed in Chapter 6.

Evidence to support the techniques of the physical examination is posted for free access by the ACP at www.acponline.org/public/bedside/. Search on any term and a list of journal articles with abstracts will be provided.

You have a patient in whom you hear an abdominal bruit. You want to read journal articles that describe what the causes may be. The following screen shots show you the lookup using *Bedside Diagnosis.*

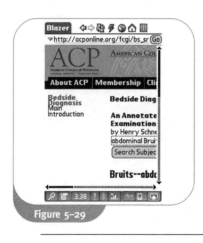

Figure 5–29

This is the home page for *Bedside Diagnosis.* On the right side you have a search box to enter the physical exam finding to be reviewed. In this example, abdominal Bruits was entered. There is a scrolling issue with this Web site and the small PDA screen. One must scroll left to right and up and down to see all the elements on the page.

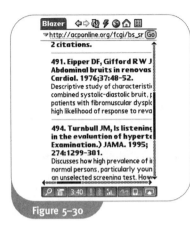

Figure 5-30

According to the screen shown here, there are two articles with abstracts on this subject.

■ Bandolier

Bandolier (www.jr2.ox.ac.uk/bandolier) is an independent journal about evidence-based health care, written by Oxford scientists and clinicians. It is printed monthly and has become the premier source of evidence-based health care information in the United Kingdom as well as worldwide for both health care professionals and consumers. Each month, PubMed and the Cochrane Library are searched for systematic reviews and meta-analyses published in the recent past. The editors at Bandolier use the latest publications to write evidence-based topical reviews.

You have a patient with recurrent migraine headaches and want to see the latest evidence-based treatments you could offer. The following screen shots demonstrate the lookup using the Bandolier Web site with a Palm PDA.

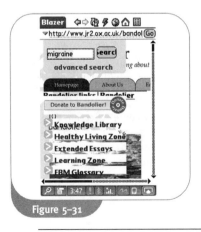

Figure 5-31

This is the home page for Bandolier. There is text overlap on the screen, but the search box is toward the top center of the page.

To demonstrate this program, enter migraine as the topic of interest and tap Search.

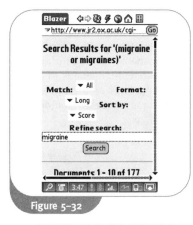

Figure 5-32

The Search Results page will allow for sorting and refinements. There are 177 topics noted for this search (this information is located at the bottom of the screen).

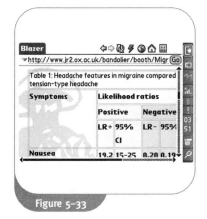

Figure 5-33

This is a table showing the likelihood ratios of symptoms that predict migraine versus tension headache.

■ Turning Research into Practice

The Turning Research into Practice (TRIP) Web site and database at www.tripdatabase.com/ is a U.K.–based search tool that allows clinicians to enter a topic in one place and have several EBM Web sites queried simultaneously.

You have a patient with recurrent migraine headaches and want to see the latest evidence-based treatments you could offer. The following screen shots demonstrate the lookup using the TRIP database Web site with a Palm PDA.

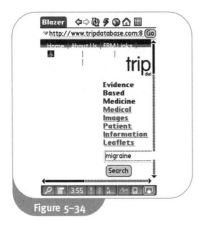

This is the home page for the TRIP database. The search box is at the bottom right of the screen. Enter migraine as your sample topic of interest, and then tap the Search button.

Figure 5-34

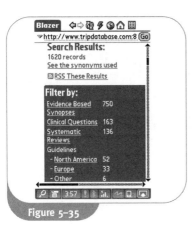

There are 1620 records found. They are categorized to allow the user to choose the desired type of article, review, or guideline.

Figure 5-35

■ The BestBETs

The BestBETs or Best Evidence Topic database at www.bestbets.org is maintained by the emergency department of the Manchester Royal Infirmary in the United Kingdom, so it is emergency focused.

You have a patient with otitis media and want to see the latest evidence-based treatments you could offer. The following screen shots demonstrate the lookup using the BestBETs Web site with a Palm PDA.

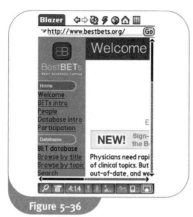

Figure 5-36

This is the home page for BestBETs. (Be careful to use .org instead of .com for the Web address, otherwise you will get a gambling Web site.)

Tap the Search option at the bottom left of the page to begin.

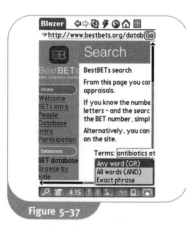

Figure 5-37

On the Search page, enter your question. As an example, antibiotics and otitis media were entered. You can choose the Boolean options of any word (OR), all words (AND), or the exact phrase you entered.

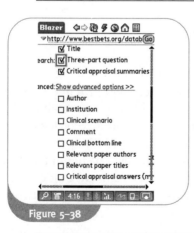

Figure 5-38

Choose the search options by tapping the appropriate checkboxes.

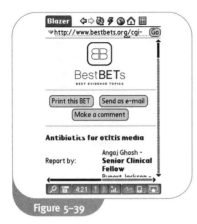

The results page is a BestBETs article.

Figure 5–39

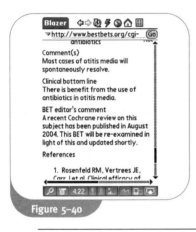

The summary has a bottom line for recommendation and references.

Figure 5–40

■ National Guideline Clearinghouse

The National Guideline Clearinghouse Web site at www.guideline.gov is a public resource for evidence-based clinical practice guidelines. NGC is an initiative of the Agency for Healthcare Research and Quality (AHRQ), U.S. Department of Health and Human Services. The editors of this site review and catalog clinical guidelines from multiple national and international health care agencies. The benefit to the user is having one authoritative site to search for relevant guidelines.

You have a patient with low back pain and want to see the latest evidence-based guidelines you could review. The following screen shots demonstrate the lookup using the NCG Web site with a Palm PDA.

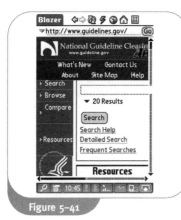

Figure 5-41

This is how the NCG Web site looks on a PDA. If you optimize the screen by turning off graphics, the text is easier to read on the screen.

Entering Back Pain in the search box and tapping Search yields the results shown in Figure 5–43.

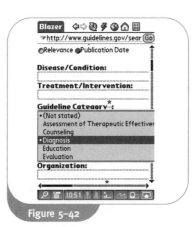

Figure 5-42

You can add limits to the search results by marking a category, such as Diagnosis.

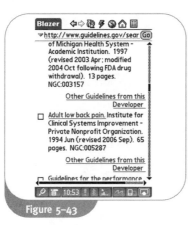

Figure 5-43

These are guidelines that you can look at by tapping on the underlined title. In this example, tap Adult low back pain.

PDA-Friendly Medical Web Sites for Clinicians ■ 89

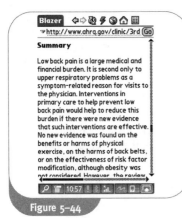

This is a summary of the guideline we obtained by tapping on Adult low back pain from the Institute for Clinical Systems Improvement.

**Summary**

Low back pain is a large medical and financial burden. It is second only to upper respiratory problems as a symptom-related reason for visits to the physician. Interventions in primary care to help prevent low back pain would help to reduce this burden if there were new evidence that such interventions are effective. No new evidence was found on the benefits or harms of physical exercise, on the harms of back belts, or on the effectiveness of risk factor modification, although obesity was not considered. However, the review

Figure 5-44

The programs described in this chapter serve as evidence that there are many helpful, free, evidence-based resources available on the Internet if you have a Web-enabled PDA. This is a powerful tool to bring the latest knowledge to patient care at the bedside.

# PDA Textbook Medical References

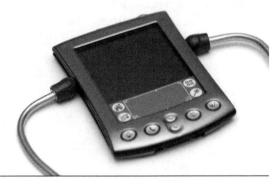

6

## Objectives

■ Discuss evidence-based electronic textbooks.

■ Review how the textbooks supplement the integrated programs.

## Why Carry Textbooks on Your PDA?

This chapter discusses popular EBM medical references available for PDAs. The power of a PDA reference is the ability to do rapid searches and the interlinks within the book. Electronic references usually come with an annual subscription for continual updates. Some are free and others have an annual fee with discounts for students and institutions. This allows your text to be current as long as you pay your subscription and regularly sync to an Internet-connected PC.

All of these references are different from the integrated software programs because they function like e-books. Some have several books, but they all may not be interlinked within topics. Different vendors use different PDA reader software, so it is beneficial to get most of your books from the same vendor. This allows the books to link to each other if the vendor did the programming. Many of these companies allow a free trial of their e-books. This is highly recommended to see how quickly the program works under clinical conditions.

# A Case to Solve

A 40-year-old male auto mechanic presents with 3 weeks of nonradiating, constant low back pain. He has been unable to work for the past week and is using heat, bed rest, and ibuprofen (200 mg every 8 hours) with very little relief. The pain began after moving some boxes at home. He has no fever, chills, weight loss, urinary flow problems, frequency, hematuria, leg weakness, numbness, or other associated symptoms. The pain is 7 out of 10 on a visual analog scale.

You want to know the best-evidence practice for diagnostic studies and treatment at this time using the these different PDA references.

■ What is the best evidence-based workup, including lab and radiological studies?

■ What is the best treatment for the most likely diagnosis?

# UpToDate

What if you had a small army of clinical experts to review all relevant clinical studies and to write detailed summaries of common primary care diseases? This is what a subscription to UpToDate provides.

UpToDate, at www.UpToDate.com, is a paid subscription service to multiple evidence-based topical reviews done by experts who synthesize the latest studies published in peer-reviewed journals and provide well-written summaries and recommendations. This is the EBM review of the literature that a clinician would be required to do to get the latest available evidence. Clinician subscribers get the online Web version, the PDA version, and the PDA Web for instant access. There is AMA category 1 CME for doing searches and reading the materials on the PC-Web version. Some PDAs with Web access may be able to search online at http://pda.UpToDate.com by entering the member's login and password.

UpToDate covers such topic specialty reviews as family medicine, pediatrics, OB-GYN, general internal medicine, and subspecialties such as cardiology, endocrinology, hematology-oncology, infectious disease, nephrology, neurology, pulmonary, critical care, and rheumatology. Upcoming reviews cover emergency medicine and allergy-immunology.

## Installation Requirements

The installation and update procedure for UpToDate on a PDA can be cumbersome. This is the only product in this book that is so large that it requires its own dedicated 2-GB memory card. You will need a Pocket PC with Windows Mobile 5.0 or 2003, Windows Pocket PC 2002, a CF or SD memory card slot with a 2-GB memory card, and a Windows-based PC with a memory card reader and DVD player.

Palm OS users need one of the following Palm devices: a Treo 650, a Treo 700p, a Palm TX with a 2-GB SD memory card, or a memory card reader linked to a Windows-based PC with a DVD drive. Palm LifeDrive users may install the entire program on the hard drive, and it does not need an SD memory card or reader.

If the PDA has Web or wireless Web capability, you can access the Web version at http://pda.UpToDate.com. Not all devices or services are validated or supported.

The following screen shots will demonstrate how you would use UpToDate to help diagnose and treat a patient with acute low back pain. A video demonstration of UpToDate, labeled Video 6–1, is available on the CD-ROM.

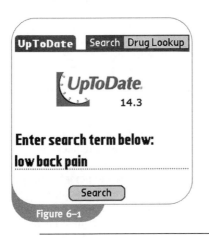

UpToDate
Search
Drug Lookup
UpToDate
14.3
Enter search term below:
low back pain
Search
Figure 6–1

To start UpToDate, place the memory card with the program in the PDA memory slot. You then can tap the icon to start the program.

This is the opening screen for UpToDate. Enter a search term on the blank line; then tap the Search button.

On the top menu is a direct link for a drug lookup. The drug reference is provided by Lexicomp.

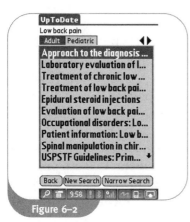
Figure 6-2

The results of the low back pain search are listed by adult or pediatric topics. You can tap on the Adult or Pediatric tab depending on the information you want. Simply tap the topic of interest. The Approach to the diagnosis of adult low back pain is selected here.

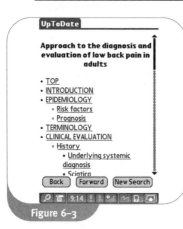
Figure 6-3

A menu of subtopics appears for fast navigation. The subtopics are listed by disease. You should have a good idea about the differential diagnosis before looking up diseases. The descriptions are extensive and well researched, but not quick summaries.

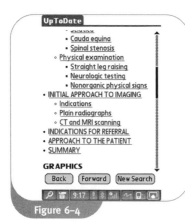
Figure 6-4

The remainder of the submenu includes history details and alarm symptoms that point to the most harmful diagnoses. These are helpful to know when formulating the workup, deciding which patient might need further diagnostic studies.

Tap on Alarm symptoms underneath History.

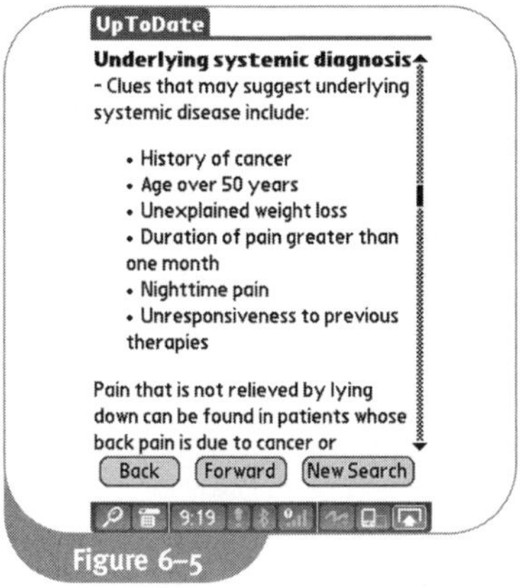

**Underlying systemic diagnosis**
- Clues that may suggest underlying systemic disease include:

- History of cancer
- Age over 50 years
- Unexplained weight loss
- Duration of pain greater than one month
- Nighttime pain
- Unresponsiveness to previous therapies

Pain that is not relieved by lying down can be found in patients whose back pain is due to cancer or

[ Back ] [ Forward ] [ New Search ]

9:19

**Figure 6–5**

Tapping Alarm symptoms gives a review of symptoms that may suggest neoplasm or infection. There are highlighted reference numbers that you may tap and see.

---

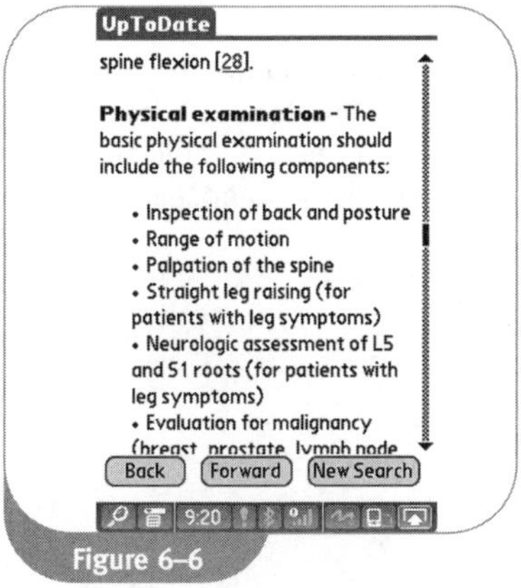

UpToDate

spine flexion [28].

**Physical examination** - The basic physical examination should include the following components:

- Inspection of back and posture
- Range of motion
- Palpation of the spine
- Straight leg raising (for patients with leg symptoms)
- Neurologic assessment of L5 and S1 roots (for patients with leg symptoms)
- Evaluation for malignancy (breast, prostate, lymph node

[ Back ] [ Forward ] [ New Search ]

9:20

**Figure 6–6**

The physical examination findings, special maneuvers, and diagnostic studies make up the next section.

---

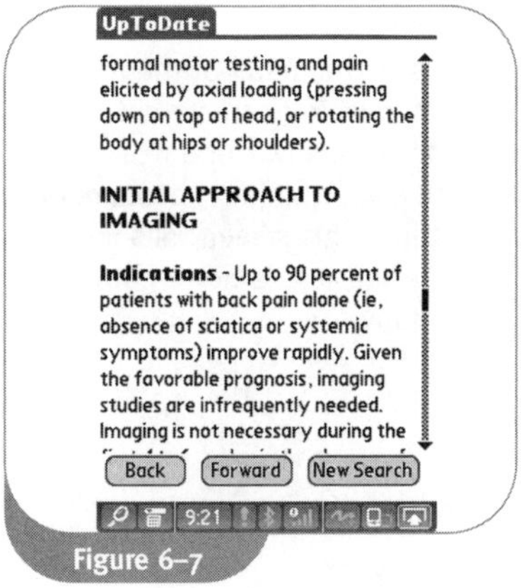

UpToDate

formal motor testing, and pain elicited by axial loading (pressing down on top of head, or rotating the body at hips or shoulders).

**INITIAL APPROACH TO IMAGING**

**Indications** - Up to 90 percent of patients with back pain alone (ie, absence of sciatica or systemic symptoms) improve rapidly. Given the favorable prognosis, imaging studies are infrequently needed. Imaging is not necessary during the

[ Back ] [ Forward ] [ New Search ]

9:21

**Figure 6–7**

You are interested in knowing if low back X-rays would be helpful in the diagnosis of your patient. The next few panels tell you that they would not be helpful.

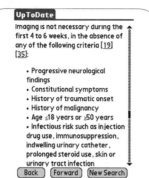

Figure 6–8

Note the underlined numbers 19 and 35 in this figure. They are highlighted references to support the recommendations. You may click on these numbers to go to the reference to which they correspond.

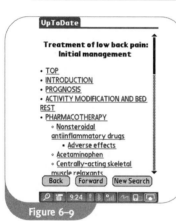

Figure 6–9

This screen shows the treatment menu for acute low back pain. Tap on any topic and detailed text will appear.

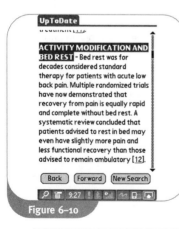

Figure 6–10

This is the detail of the non-pharmacologic treatment. You want to know if bed rest or activity is the best recommendation. This screen tells you that bed rest is not a good therapy.

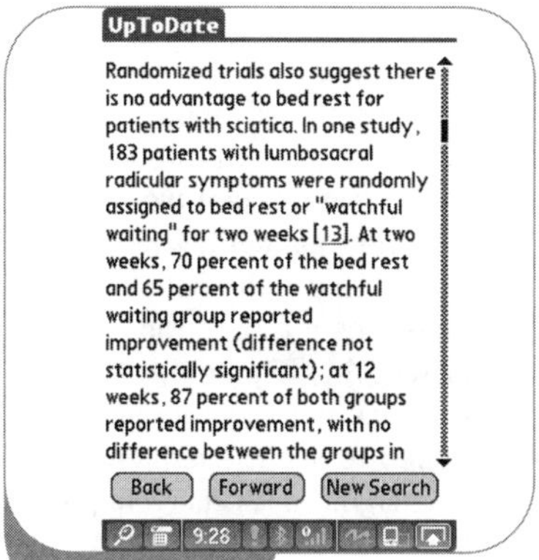

**UpToDate**

Randomized trials also suggest there
is no advantage to bed rest for
patients with sciatica. In one study,
183 patients with lumbosacral
radicular symptoms were randomly
assigned to bed rest or "watchful
waiting" for two weeks [13]. At two
weeks, 70 percent of the bed rest
and 65 percent of the watchful
waiting group reported
improvement (difference not
statistically significant); at 12
weeks, 87 percent of both groups
reported improvement, with no
difference between the groups in

[ Back ] [ Forward ] [ New Search ]

🔍 📷 9:28 ⧖ ⚡ 📶 📧 🖥️ 📷

**Figure 6–11**

You learn that there would be a quicker recovery if you keep your patient active.

---

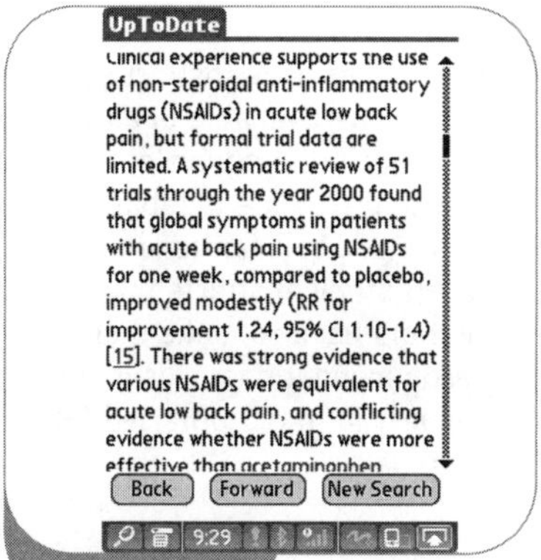

**UpToDate**

Clinical experience supports the use
of non-steroidal anti-inflammatory
drugs (NSAIDs) in acute low back
pain, but formal trial data are
limited. A systematic review of 51
trials through the year 2000 found
that global symptoms in patients
with acute back pain using NSAIDs
for one week, compared to placebo,
improved modestly (RR for
improvement 1.24, 95% CI 1.10-1.4)
[15]. There was strong evidence that
various NSAIDs were equivalent for
acute low back pain, and conflicting
evidence whether NSAIDs were more
effective than acetaminophen

[ Back ] [ Forward ] [ New Search ]

🔍 📷 9:29 ⧖ ⚡ 📶 📧 🖥️ 📷

**Figure 6–12**

In the treatment section, there are links to medication details if you tap on the highlighted name. The drug database is very comprehensive and is provided by Lexicomp.

---

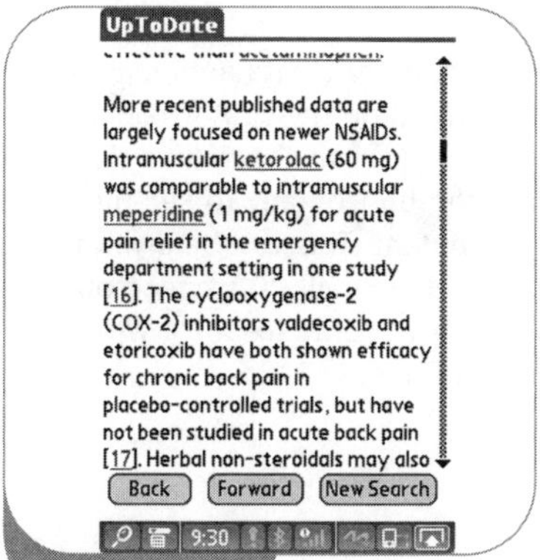

**UpToDate**

effective than acetaminophen.

More recent published data are
largely focused on newer NSAIDs.
Intramuscular ketorolac (60 mg)
was comparable to intramuscular
meperidine (1 mg/kg) for acute
pain relief in the emergency
department setting in one study
[16]. The cyclooxygenase-2
(COX-2) inhibitors valdecoxib and
etoricoxib have both shown efficacy
for chronic back pain in
placebo-controlled trials, but have
not been studied in acute back pain
[17]. Herbal non-steroidals may also

[ Back ] [ Forward ] [ New Search ]

🔍 📷 9:30 ⧖ ⚡ 📶 📧 🖥️ 📷

**Figure 6–13**

More about treatment options is provided, answering common clinical questions with evidence from current studies.

---

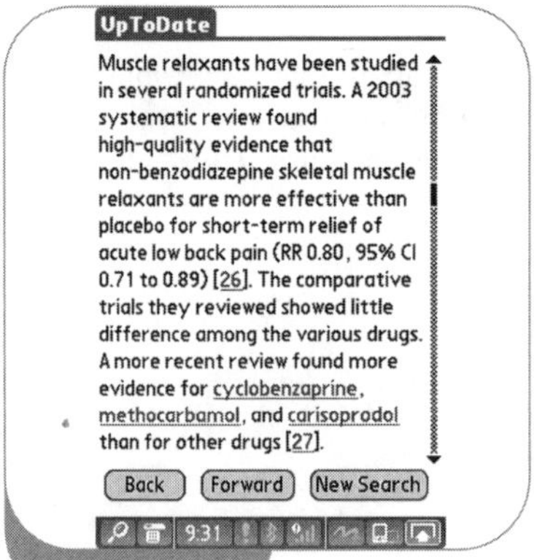

UpToDate
Muscle relaxants have been studied in several randomized trials. A 2003 systematic review found high-quality evidence that non-benzodiazepine skeletal muscle relaxants are more effective than placebo for short-term relief of acute low back pain (RR 0.80, 95% CI 0.71 to 0.89) [26]. The comparative trials they reviewed showed little difference among the various drugs. A more recent review found more evidence for cyclobenzaprine, methocarbamol, and carisoprodol than for other drugs [27].
Back
Forward
New Search
9:31

Figure 6–14

This screen is found while scrolling through the treatment text. You want to know if a muscle relaxant would help the treatment. A review of the topic with abstracted references provides the answer. Any highlighted reference number can be tapped to see the reference, as in Figure 6–15. Each highlighted medication links to detailed information.

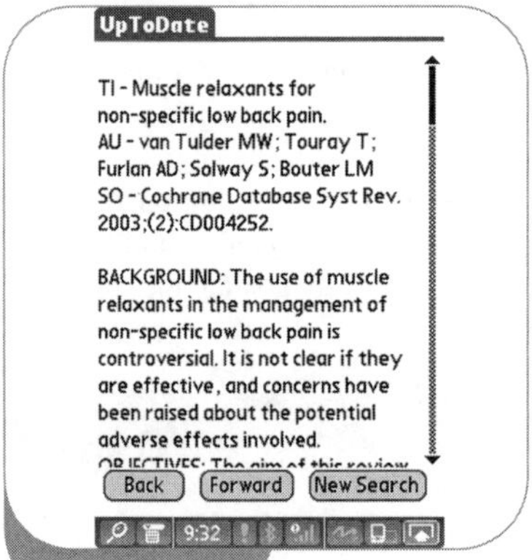

UpToDate
TI - Muscle relaxants for non-specific low back pain.
AU - van Tulder MW; Touray T; Furlan AD; Solway S; Bouter LM
SO - Cochrane Database Syst Rev. 2003;(2):CD004252.
BACKGROUND: The use of muscle relaxants in the management of non-specific low back pain is controversial. It is not clear if they are effective, and concerns have been raised about the potential adverse effects involved.
Back
Forward
New Search
9:32

Figure 6–15

References with abstract summaries are available in all topics. This is the equivalent of a selected Medline database in your PDA. You can read the latest study abstracts that the authors used to make their recommendations. This is the highest form of appraised EBM materials.

UpToDate
The spinal unit
Disc
Nucleus pulposus
Vertebra
The spinal unit consists of a three-jo
comprising two posterior apophysea
articulations and the vertebral body
Back
Forward
New Search
9:34

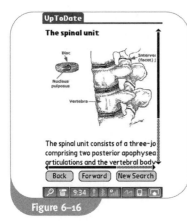

Figure 6–16

There are charts and images stored on the PDA version. The user must scroll vertically and horizontally to see the content. This can be awkward on the small PDA screen but is a valuable resource when bedside.

It is the author's opinion that UpToDate is one of the best and most comprehensive EBM e-book references you can buy for primary care. It is not quick to use because of the comprehensive materials and sub-menu structure, but is an excellent complement to the quick integrated programs recommended throughout this book. In addition, there are options for CME credits. The limitations of the program include the necessity of a separate 2-GB memory card to be placed in your PDA, and the detailed content that requires more than a few minutes to get your answers.

## BMJ Clinical Evidence

BMJ Clinical Evidence at www.clinicalevidence.org is a paid subscription service from the editors of the BMJ Publishing Group. This PDA e-book is a full copy of the biyearly updated *BMJ Clinical Evidence* paperback books and Web site with the same content. The PDA version is packaged using the Unbound Medicine reader, the same reader for the Merck*Medicus* e-books. There is a free trial version to download at www.clinicalevidence.org/ceweb/products/PDA.jsp. There are several review articles of common clinical topics in primary care.

The following screen shots will demonstrate how you would use the BMJ Clinical Evidence service to help manage a patient with acute low back pain. A video demonstration of BMJ Clinical Evidence, labeled Video 6–2, is available on the CD-ROM.

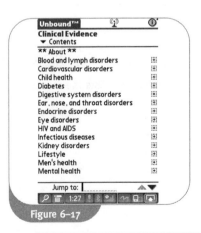

This is the main menu page that is displayed when you tap the CE icon on your PDA. You can change from a body system listing to a topical one by tapping on the Contents drop-down menu.

Figure 6–17

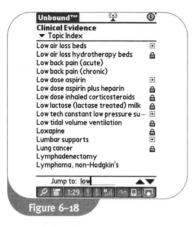

Figure 6-18

This is the Topic Index. There is a Jump to function at the bottom of the screen to enter your key words for a search.

You are interested in low back pain, so you type in the word "low." After entering the word, you see the topics beginning with Low come up, including acute and chronic low back pain. You then tap on Low back pain (acute) for a review of the subject.

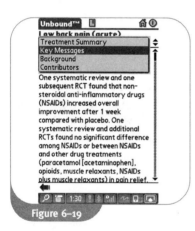

Figure 6-19

The Treatment Summary is a list of all treatment modalities, including pharmacologic, non-pharmacologic, and surgical. The benefits of each are discussed with the evidence.

Key messages are summaries of the main points of treatment and diagnosis.

Background discusses the pathophysiology, incidence, etiology, prognosis, aims, outcomes, and methods used to review the medical literature.

Contributors lists the article's authors.

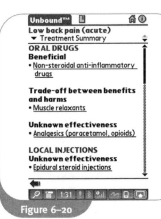

Figure 6–20

Medications are listed by class and are linked to additional details if you tap on the underlined word. Specific drug information, however, is not provided, so you must use another resource.

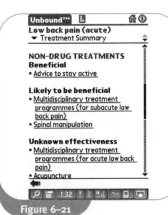

Figure 6–21

The nondrug treatments recommend staying active. You want to know more about why, so you tap the highlighted text.

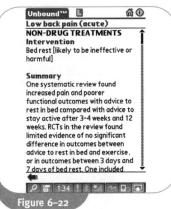

Figure 6–22

A referenced review is displayed giving the best evidence for the recommendation. This provides a quick resource of appraised evidence.

In summary, BMJ Clinical Evidence is a quick, inexpensive, and informative PDA reference for students and clinicians. It covers many common topics seen in primary care.

## InfoRetriever and InfoPOEMs

InfoRetriever and InfoPOEMs (Patient Oriented Evidence that Matters) at www.infopoems.com is a paid subscription service from John Wiley & Sons. First established by primary care physicians, this is a PDA reference with evidence-based ranked summaries of several journal articles' practice guidelines and the 5-Minute Clinical Consult. There is Web site access for Web-connected PCs and PDAs that is accessible with the subscription and a daily e-mail POEM. CME credits are offered for many searches.

The following screen shots will demonstrate how you would use InfoRetriever to help manage a patient with acute low back pain.

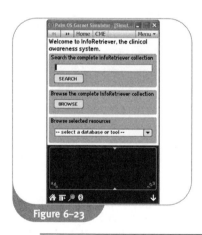

This is the opening screen after tapping the InfoRetriever icon. You start by entering a search term and selecting the type of search.

Figure 6–23

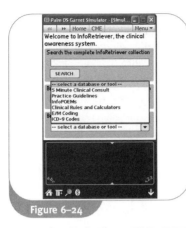

Figure 6–24

The types of search options are listed in a drop-down menu when you tap on the down arrow under Browse selected resources in Figure 6–23. Select any word to search all of the stored resources.

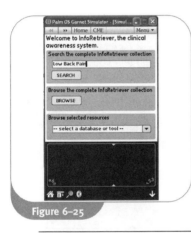

Figure 6–25

Enter low back pain as the search term in the first box and tap Search.

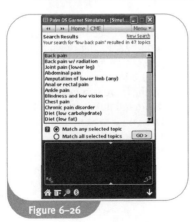

Figure 6–26

The resulting diseases or symptoms appear in a list for you to choose. Tap Back pain.

Palm OS Garnet Simulator - [Simul...
Home
CME
Menu
Search Results
New Search
Your topic selection produced 96 results
-- refine by type of result --
-- refine by type of resource --
Acupuncture effective for chronic bac...
Acupuncture for low back pain (LOE = 1...
Acute low back pain (UMHS) (LOE = 1a)
Adult low back pain (ICSI) (LOE = 1a)
Antidepressants beneficial in some wit...
Back belts to prevent occ'l back pain (...
Back pain evaluation guideline (LOE = 1a)
Back schools for non-specific low back...
Page: 1 2 3 4 5 6 7 8

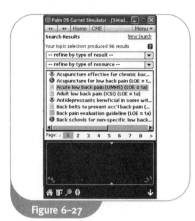

Figure 6–27

Tapping Acute low back pain (UMHS) will open the practice guidelines in Figure 6–28.

Palm OS Garnet Simulator - [Simul...
Home
CME
Menu
Treatment Guideline: Acute low back pain
Reference: University of Michigan Health System. Acute low back pain. Ann Arbor (MI): University of Michigan Health System; 2003 Apr. 13 p.
Acute low back pain
University of Michigan Health System - Academic Institution
Released: 1997 (revised 2003 Apr; modified 2004 Oct following FDA drug withdrawal)

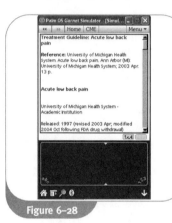

Figure 6–28

Tapping Acute low back pain (UMHS) (seen in the previous figures) lets you read the guideline shown here.

You must read through all the guidelines and choose the one that is best suited for your patient.

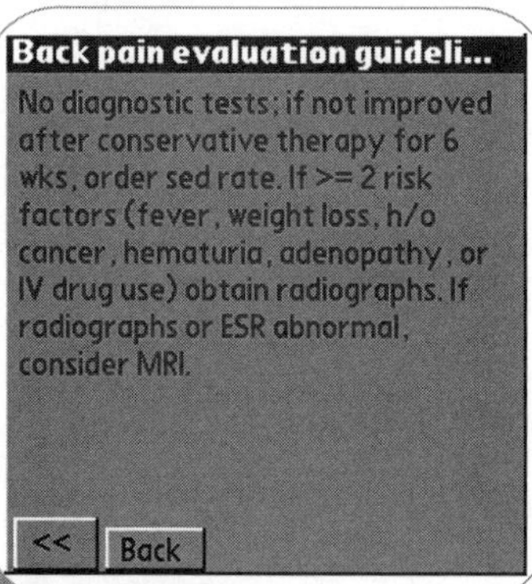

Back pain evaluation guideli...
No diagnostic tests; if not improved after conservative therapy for 6 wks, order sed rate. If >= 2 risk factors (fever, weight loss, h/o cancer, hematuria, adenopathy, or IV drug use) obtain radiographs. If radiographs or ESR abnormal, consider MRI.
<<
Back

Figure 6–29

Tapping on Decision Support, found by scrolling down the main search menu, (Figure 6–26) brings you to this screen. There is a unique feature in InfoRetriever that gives you a capsule summary of all the diagnostic recommendations.

Overall, InfoRetriever is a collection of the latest references, practice guidelines, and decision support rules. Its searches can be slow and difficult, because you must sort through all the different choices.

## *Mobile* Merck*Medicus* and the *Merck Manual*

This is currently a free service after completing a registration at www.merckmedicus.com/pp/us/hcp/templates/tier2/PDAtools.jsp, and it is recommended for all clinicians and students. Licensed providers should choose their professional category and enter their state license. The PDA structure is provided by Unbound Medicine (www.unboundmedicine.com), supplier of the free *Diagnosaurus*. Student or licensed provider status will determine the Web services provided. All of the PDA tools should be provided to students and providers alike. There is a medical student category, but not a specific PA or NP student category listed. All other students should choose the medical student category and put in a number (real or made up) in the "Other License Number" box and specify "Student ID" in the "Other License" type box. This should allow access to all of the PDA tools, but not all of the Web site tools reserved for licensed providers.

This PDA version gives free updates to the professional edition of the *Merck Manual*. The classic medical textbook is cross-linked to the other free textbook, *Pocket Guide to Diagnostic Tests*. Periodic updates flow automatically to the PDA wirelessly or when you synch to a PC that has Internet access.

*Harrison's Practice—Answers on Demand* is another classic synopsis of *Harrison's Principles and Practice of Medicine* that is excellent for fast lookups.

*Pocket Guide to Diagnostic Tests* provides evidence-based information on the selection and interpretation of over 350 laboratory, imaging, and microbiology tests.

Reuters Medical News is a news service that features top current medical news stories.

Medline Journal Abstracts are citations and abstracts for the current issue of over 200 medical journals that are searchable on Medline. You are first provided with a selection of available journals that may be of more interest to your specialty. You then have the option of editing your journal list as you wish.

For Merck*Medicus* and Medline Search, the search function on *Mobile* Merck*Medicus* is designed to let you send a request from your

PDA for a search to be run on either the Merck*Medicus* Web site or on Medline. Search results will be accessible via your Web browser the next time you synchronize your device. This allows busy clinicians to enter questions during the course of a day and then get relevant information automatically from some of the top medical resources, including Harrison's Online and *Cecil Textbook of Medicine*. Simply enter your request on your PDA, and the next time it is synchronized it will automatically run your search and make the results available to you in your *Mobile* Merck*Medicus* Record Library on the Web.

For RSS News Feeds, choose from 18 RSS feeds from the FDA, World Health Organization, National Institute of Health, and AAAS Eureka to add to your device.

There are several other full-text online references and services available with a Web-enabled PDA.

The following screen shots will demonstrate how you would use *Mobile* Merck*Medicus* to help manage a patient with acute low back pain. A video demonstration of *Mobile* Merck*Medicus,* labeled Video 6–3, is available on the CD-ROM.

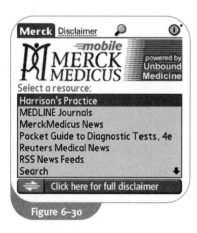

Figure 6–30

This is the main menu for the *Mobile* Merck*Medicus* product. Choose a book, then do a search. The search function on this menu will search the Merck*Medicus* Web site the next time you are synced or linked to the Web. It does not do a global search of the PDA resources.

The main disease resources are *Harrison's Practice* and the *Merck Manual.*

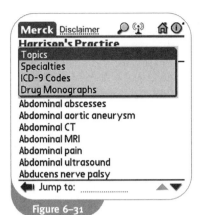

Figure 6-31

Tap on *Harrison's Practice* (as shown in Figure 6–30) and see a menu that can be displayed by topics, specialties, ICD-9 codes, or drugs.

In the Jump to blank, enter back pain and tap that topic.

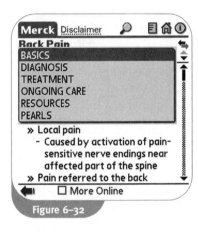

Figure 6-32

Each topic is arranged with the following subheadings:

Basics: the pathophysiology and related anatomy of back pain

Diagnosis: the history, physical examination, differential diagnosis, lab tests, and imaging studies

Treatment: pharmacologic and nonpharmacologic treatments

Ongoing Care: monitoring, referral, prognosis, prevention, and complications

Resources: ICD-9 codes, Web sites, and references

Pearls: clinical summary statements for quick review

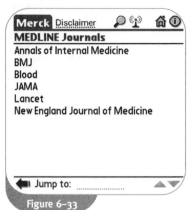

From the main menu (Figure 6–30), tap MEDLINE Journals to see a list. Tap any journal and see the table of contents for the latest issue.

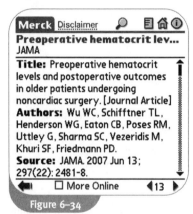

Tap on an article title to see an abstract for a quick reading, as shown on this screen. This is an easy way to keep current with the latest major medical journals.

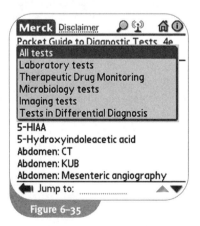

From the main menu (Figure 6–30), tap the Pocket Guide to Diagnostic Tests, 4e to review lab and imaging studies. This has imaging tests that are not present in the Epocrates Lab section.

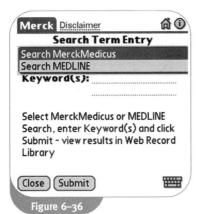

Figure 6-36

From the main menu (Figure 6-30), tap the Search option. Search will allow you to enter a search that will provide a list of responses on the Merck*Medicus* Web site after you sync.

You can construct the search while seeing patients, but the answer will not come until you sync later.

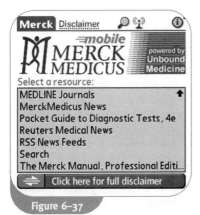

Figure 6-37

Go back to the main menu; the last resource listed is the *Merck Manual,* Professional Edition.

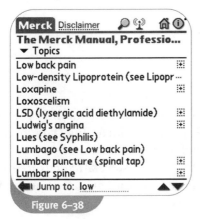

Figure 6-38

This classic e-book is arranged by topics or sections (body systems). To get to your current topic of interest, enter "low" in the Jump to blank and see the topic list (as shown in this figure), including Low back pain. Tap on this to get to the text.

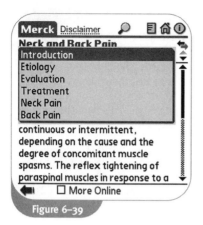

Each topic chapter has an introduction, etiology, evaluation, and treatment section that you can navigate to using the drop-down menu.

Figure 6–39

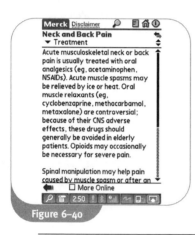

The *Merck Manual* reads like an e-book with some topical links to other books within the suite. To see the existing links, tap the red and blue horizontal arrows next to the topic title and a list will appear. Tapping the link will take you to the related text in the included books.

Figure 6–40

Unbound Medicine at www.unboundmedicine.com offers several other PDA books by McGraw-Hill Professional, including *Diagnosaurus 2.0,* a free differential diagnosis tool for the Web and PDA.

It is the author's opinion that the *Mobile* Merck*Medicus* free PDA product is a must-have reference for every student and clinician. It is quick, efficient, and has excellent resources.

## Medicine Central

In addition to providing the Merck*Medicus* free PDA book collection and the paid subscription for BMJ Clinical Evidence, Unbound Medicine (www.unboundmedicine.com) offers several PDA books and bundles for sale. There are several "central" bundles, such as medicine, pediatrics, anesthesia, emergency, that combine excellent textbooks with drug references, *Diagnosaurus,* and journal abstracts. These texts have some links established to jump books to related topics, but not extensive hyperlinks as described in the integrated PDA products covered in Chapter 4. You can purchase well-known PDA textbooks that run in a familiar and stable reader if you use the *Mobile* Merck*Medicus* suite of programs.

The following figures show the Medicine Central product with the 5-Minute Clinical Consult, *Diagnosaurus,* and *Davis's Drug Guide, Pocket Guide to Diagnostic Tests,* and Unbound Medline. You also may choose *Harrison's Manual of Medicine* or *Current Consult Medicine* as the main medical text instead of the 5-Minute Clinical Consult/ *Diagnosaurus* combination. Options are available for wireless Black-Berry and iPhone users.

The following screen shots will demonstrate how you would use Medicine Central to help manage a patient with acute low back pain. A video demonstration of Medicine Central, labeled Video 6–4, is available on the CD-ROM.

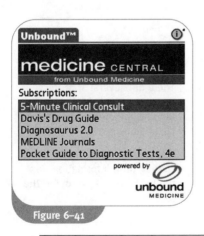

Figure 6–41

This is the opening page for Medicine Central. The books you see on the menu have some links.

*Diagnosaurus* is the same book available for free as described in Chapter 3.

Medline and *Pocket Guide to Diagnostic Tests, 4e* are the same features in the free Merck*Medicus* suite.

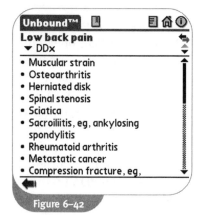

Figure 6–42

Tap on *Diagnosaurus* and enter low back pain to view the differential diagnosis. Tap on the red and blue horizontal arrows in the right upper corner to open the link box.

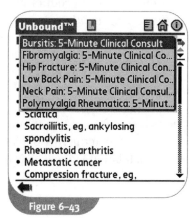

Figure 6–43

These are the book links available to take you to related text in the 5-Minute Clinical Consult. All of the listed differential diagnoses do not have corresponding one-to-one links.

Tap on Low Back Pain.

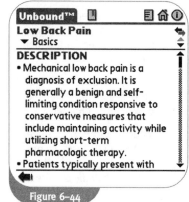

Figure 6–44

This is the 5-Minute Clinical Consult text for Low Back Pain. There are several subtopics that you can navigate to by tapping the menu down arrow next to basics.

To see the related links, including drug information, tap the red/blue links arrow at the top.

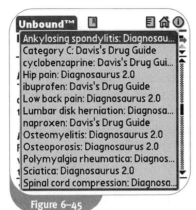

Figure 6-45

These are the related links in *Davis's Drug Guide* and back to the differential diagnosis list in *Diagnosaurus*.

Tap naproxen to see specific drug information.

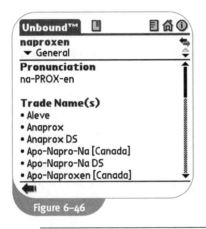

Figure 6-46

This is the drug information screen in *Davis's Drug Guide* for naproxen. To see the subtopic navigation menu, tap the down arrow next to General, under the drug title.

It is the author's opinion that the cost of Medicine Central may be better spent on a fully integrated product along with the free Merck*Medicus* and *Diagnosaurus* products from Unbound Medicine. If you need references for other specialties like pediatrics, anesthesia, or emergency medicine, the Central Series may be what you need. Unbound Medicine also allows Web access to your subscription using a PC or your Web-enabled PDA. The installation, updating, and program navigation features are all excellent.

# Clinical Xpert

Clinical Xpert is a free PDA reference from Thomson, the publishers of the *Physician Desk Reference* (*PDR*) and the Micromedex series. You must fill out an online registration at www.thomsonclinicalxpert.com and identify yourself as a prescribing clinician or student. You also can register at www.PDR.net.

Included are a medical test; drug- and drug-interaction references; information on alternative medicine, labs, and toxicology; medical calculators; and medical news. For a free reference, this is a wonderful resource for students and practicing clinicians. The toxicology feature is unique and a wonderful resource for those working in emergency medicine. The other e-books are nice complements to the integrated software everyone should have.

The following screen shots will demonstrate how you would use Clinical Xpert to help manage a patient with acute low back pain. A video demonstration of Clinical Xpert labeled Video 6–5 is available on the CD-ROM.

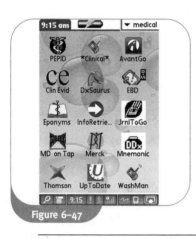

The program icon is the four-pronged star with Thomson underneath.

Figure 6–47

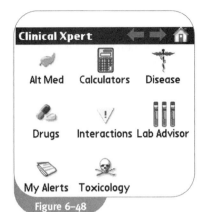

Figure 6-48

The main menu shows the available sections. This is very much like the paid programs, but the content is geared to the drug/toxicology content. (Remember, this is the *PDR* and Micromedex authors.)

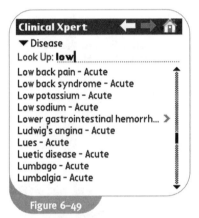

Figure 6-49

Click on Disease to see an alphabetical index. You can get to your subject quickly by entering the first few letters.

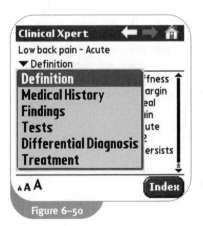

Figure 6-50

Each disease section is divided into six sections that can be navigated by tapping on the drop-down box. The "All sections" option will show the content, and you can scroll down through each section.

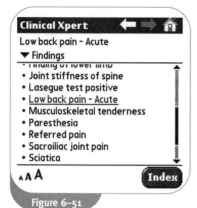

Any underlined-highlighted item will be hyperlinked to that subject. However, there are not many links within the text.

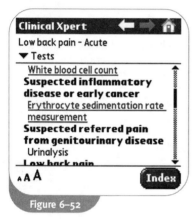

Highlighted and underlined tests are linked to the lab section with details.

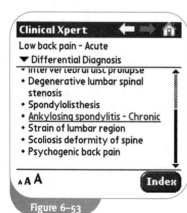

This program has a limited number of links to other diseases in the reference. About one out of nine diseases is hyperlinked.

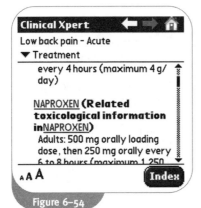

Figure 6–54

There are extensive drug and toxicology links. This is where the Clinical Xpert content excels.

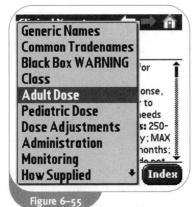

Figure 6–55

Extensive drug information can be accessed from the drop-down menu that appears as an arrow next to Treatment in Figure 6–54. This is a nice complement to the integrated software.

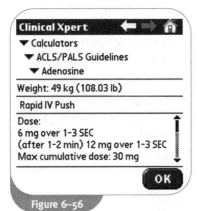

Figure 6–56

Choosing the calculator function from the main menu (Figure 6–48) allows you to choose adult or pediatric dose, and offers you a line to enter weight. The calculator computes the correct ACLS/PALS drug dose for commonly used medications.

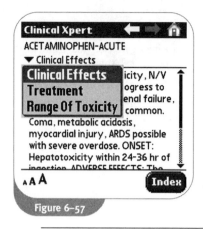

Choosing the Toxicology function from the main menu (Figure 6–48) allows you to review the management details for drug overdoses, like acetaminophen. This feature is unique and not found in any other bundle. It is recommended for anyone working in emergency medicine.

Figure 6–57

In the author's opinion, as a free resource, this is a recommended reference for all students and clinicians. It offers some unique e-books on toxicology and alternative medicine. Because it is from the makers of the *PDR* and Micromedix, the drug and toxicology information is extensive and complements the integrated programs.

## DynaMed

DynaMed at www.dynamicmedical.com is a clinical reference tool created by physicians for physicians and other health care professionals for use primarily at the point of care. It contains clinically organized summaries for nearly 2000 topics. Based on the results of a study published in the *Annals of Family Medicine* (2005), not only did primary care clinicians answer more clinical questions with access to DynaMed than without DynaMed, but these clinicians also found more answers in DynaMed that changed clinical decisions.

The disease summary sections are:

■ Description (including ICD-9 codes): subcategories include definition, applicable ICD-9 codes, types, organs involved, who is most affected, and incidence or prevalence

■ Causes and Risk Factors: subcategories include causes, pathogenesis, likely risk factors, possible risk factors, and factors not associated with increased risk

■ Complications and Associated Conditions: subcategories include disease complications and other problems that may accompany it

- History: subcategories include chief complaint, history of present illness, meds, past medical history, family history, social history, and review of systems; these categories currently use the standard shortcut codes used by U.S.-based care providers in patient charts (e.g., CC, FH, PH, Meds, etc.); because these codes are not standard beyond the United States, DynaMed will change these to the full terms and phrases
- Physical: subcategories include general physical; skin; head, eyes, ears, nose, and throat (HEENT); neck; chest; cardiac; lungs; abdomen; back; extremities; neurological; rectal; pelvic; and miscellaneous physical
- Diagnosis: subcategories include making the diagnosis, rule out, tests to order, blood tests, urine studies, imaging studies, CKG, CSF analysis, pathology tests, and other diagnostic testing
- Prognosis: describes the likelihood of recovery or potential for death
- Treatment: subcategories include treatment overview, diet, activity, counseling, medications, surgery, consultation and referral, other management, and follow-up
- Prevention and Screening: describes prevention measures and lists general screening tools that can detect the disease at an early stage
- References: subcategories include general references used, reviews, and guidelines
- Patient Information: describes patient education information that can be shared about the disease
- Acknowledgments: subcategories include author, maintainer, and reviewer information

Each disease summary has numerous hyperlinks to public access electronic journal articles and practice guidelines, as well as to a few key subscription-based resources (e.g., Cochrane Library, Medical Letter).

DynaMed's staff monitors more than 100 journals daily. An additional 400 journals are monitored through journal-review services along with systematic reviews, guidelines, and drug information sources. Information added as a result of this literature surveillance is noted at the top of the respective disease summaries and includes the update date and the section to which it was incorporated. Topics included in the database may be reorganized or new topics added in response to new evidence.

The following screen shots will demonstrate how you would use DynaMed to help manage a patient with acute low back pain. A video demonstration of DynaMed, labeled Video 6–6, is available on the CD-ROM.

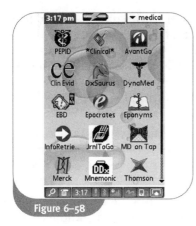

Figure 6-58

Click on the DynaMed caduceus to start the program. The program uses the Skyscape reader, so the opening screen will be from Skyscape.

This book will be linked to other Skyscape e-books if you choose to purchase additional titles.

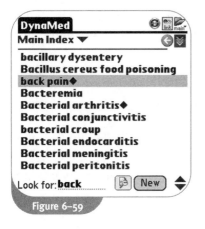

Figure 6-59

Using the Skyscape interface, DynaMed is designed to look like any Skyscape PDA book.

There is a drop-down menu with sections. Icons in the upper-right corner of the screen are:

Circle button: wireless updates

Link button: links you to any other Skyscape PDA book you have purchased; also will take you to a related topic if there is one

Folder: main index for personal notes

Back arrow: to see the last page viewed

Down arrows: help and history of views

At the bottom are search functions, New for starting a new note, and scrolling arrows.

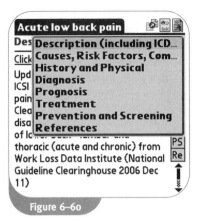

Figure 6-60

Each topic opens with the latest EBM study and date the information in the section was last updated. ICD-9 codes are provided for easy access. This is the submenu for acute low back pain. It is obtained by tapping on the drop-down menu in the upper left of the screen under Description.

There is no drug database, but classes of medications are listed in the treatment section.

There are annotated references and lists of review articles on each topic.

There is a link to other Skyscape books that will take you to chapters with the same title.

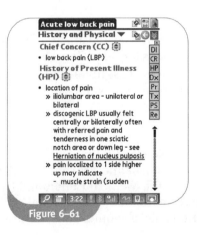

Figure 6-61

This is the History and Physical Examination screen. This has a SOAP (subjective, objective, assessment, and plan) note approach and body system approach to the Hx and PE.

The Hx and PE section describes the significance of positive findings, which is excellent for students.

There is a drop-down section heading and an abbreviated section heading on the right side of the screen for easy navigation. This is the same navigation menu for Skyscape e-books.

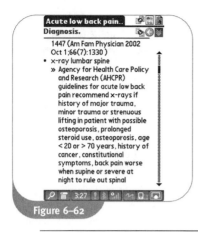

**Figure 6–62**

In the Treatment section of the menu is a referenced review of lumbar x-rays for acute low back pain. Topics are referenced with articles and guidelines. Summaries and recommendations are easy to find and are a quick read.

This reference should be considered by both students and clinicians. It offers appraised EBM summaries on many of the common primary care and emergency medicine topics. The authors have reviewed the literature, made recommendations, and summarize the best evidence in a quick and efficient program for the PDA.

## Clinical Constellation

Probably the leader in medical PDA titles, Skyscape at www.Skyscape. com offers over 400 medical PDA textbooks for sale. They offer a reader that has a consistent navigation menu and cross links between books. In addition, there are many free PDA resources such as

- Archimedes, a medical calculator
- ACC Pocket Guidelines
- 911, an emergency management resource that incorporates content from the Centers for Disease Control and Prevention (CDC), World Health Organization (WHO), the Medical Letter, and Outlines in Clinical Medicine to provide medical professionals with the latest information on infectious disease outbreaks, natural disasters, and bioterrorism threats
- MedStream 360°, medical information channels, a collection of medical information channels that keep you up to date on a broad range of journal articles, medical news, and research studies

■ Skyscape CME 360°, a convenient and flexible way to fulfill CME requirements

■ Skyscape Food Guide, a handy handheld tool to help educate patients on choosing foods and the correct amounts

■ MedAlert, delivers the latest medical information and breaking news by specialty directly to your PDA

■ CheckRx, a drug interactions guide that helps keep patients safe and informed about adverse drug interactions

Skyscape Clinical Constellation at www.skyscape.com/estore/ ProductDetail.aspx?ProductId=1180 and www.skyscape.com/group/ GroupHome.aspx is a bundle of clinical books with some interlinked text. This does not function like the integrated software, but it is a collection of excellent references if you do not wish to use the integrated programs discussed in Chapter 3.

The following screen shots will demonstrate how you would use Clinical Constellation to help manage a patient with acute low back pain.

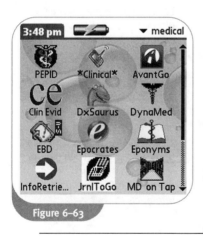

Figure 6–63

*Clinical* is the icon for Clinical Constellation. The installation program may put it in a new Skyscape grouping on your PDA. You can change this and add it to your medical group as described in the video.

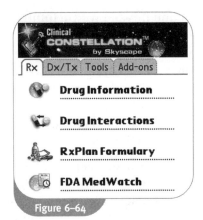

This is the main menu with the different categories of e-books. Across the top in order are:

Rx: Drug references

Dx/Tx: Diagnostic and treatment

Tools: Medical calculators

Add-ons: The extras

Figure 6–64

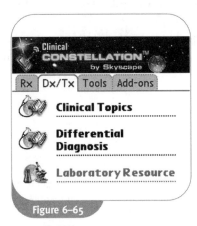

Clinical Topics is the 5-Minute Clinical Consult text discussed in Chapter 4.

Differential Diagnosis is Mobile DDx by Zeiger and Doherty. This is the same text available for free as *Diagnosaurus* discussed in Chapter 3.

Laboratory Resources is an additional reference book that you can order, but is not included in this package. The link does not work unless you add the book.

Figure 6–65

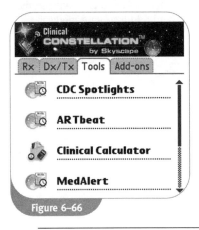

There are tools such as CDC Spotlights, ART beat with news updates, a clinical calculator, MedAlert, and (when you scroll down) an ICD-9 lookup reference.

Figure 6–66

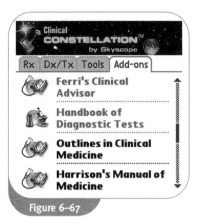

Figure 6-67

The Add-ons section is a list of recommended PDA textbooks, each at an additional annual price from Skyscape.

Skyscape has a large collection of PDA textbooks that are cross-linked to go from one book to another.

*Harrison's* full text does not come in Constellation, but it will be reviewed as part of this package. It must be purchased separately from Skyscape.

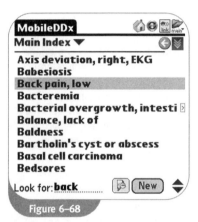

Figure 6-68

This screen is the index of MobileDDx. This is the same text as the free *Diagnosaurus* discussed in Chapter 3.

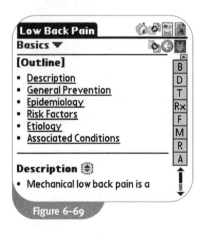

Figure 6-69

This screen is the Basics page for acute low back pain within the 5-Minute Clinical Consult. There is a list of submenu topics and a sidebar menu.

B—Basics

D—Diagnosis and DDx

T—Treatments

Rx—Medications

F—Follow-up

M—Miscellaneous and ICD-9 codes

R—References

A—Author

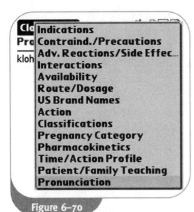

Figure 6-70

Tapping on Drug Information in Figure 6–64 brings you to a reference text with these sections listed for any drug chosen.

This can be found in the recommended integrated software and the free e-books.

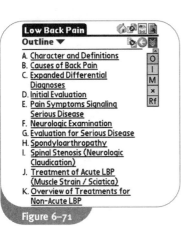

Figure 6-71

Tapping on Outlines in Clinical Medicine (Figure 6–67) opens this screen. This is a reference that has appraised evidence and concise recommendations. The sections for Low Back Pain are listed, and the right side box menu is the same for most topics.

O—Outline: an overview of the topic with the differential diagnosis and work-up

I—Information, including overview, causes, workup, and recommended diagnostic tests, all referenced and hyperlinked to the reference title

M—Medications

x—No material for this subject

Rf—Resources and References

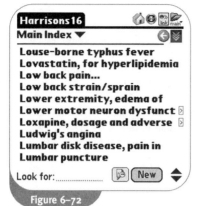

Figure 6-72

Tapping on *Harrison's Manual of Medicine* (Figure 6–67) brings you to this screen. The full text opens with a main index that also can display a drug index by tapping the drop-down menu.

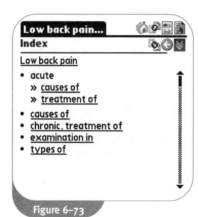

Figure 6-73

The Low back pain reference has the submenu as shown.

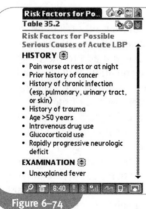

Figure 6-74

There are tables that summarize the history and physical exam for quick reference.

It is the author's opinion that this is a trusted, comprehensive medical e-book that stands on its own. It can complement the recommended integrated programs.

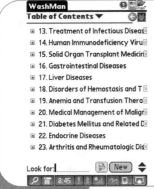

Figure 6-75

The *Washington Manual* is another classic internal medicine text reference. This can be opened from the Clinical Constellation's main menu (Figure 6–64) if you made the extra purchase. The table of contents can be viewed by disease- or topic-oriented menu.

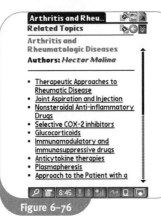

Figure 6-76

Back pain is not found in the topic search, but you can get some helpful treatment information by opening the Arthritis and Rheumatologic Disease chapter. The *Washington Manual* has general internal medicine topics and diseases and an inpatient medicine slant.

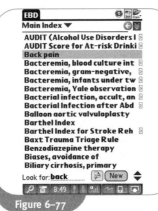

Figure 6-77

*Evidence-Based Diagnosis* is an add-on PDA textbook from Skyscape that you can purchase and add to the Clinical Constellation. If you made the extra purchase, you would enter the book from the main menu (Figure 6–64). This reference offers appraised topic reviews. This screen shows the main index. Searching for back pain, you would enter "back" on the Look for: blank and see this menu.

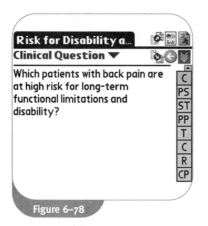

Figure 6-78

Tapping on Back pain from the index in Figure 6–77 brings you to this screen, which shows a related clinical question. The Back pain topic has a drop-down and right-sided box menu for fast navigation.

The topic is posed like a PICO question and then answered with evidence from one or more studies.

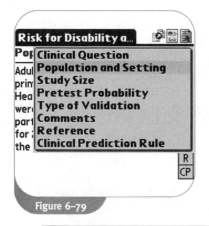

Figure 6-79

Tapping on the drop-down menu opens this submenu. This evidence-based resource is not comprehensive and does not offer details regarding workup, treatment, or prevention. It may help answer specific clinical questions. This does not provide enough clinical depth for use in the 2- to 3-minute "tell me what I need to know" mode.

Overall, it is the author's opinion that Clinical Constellation is not as good as the recommended integrated programs and free e-books that offer the same information in a faster, easier-to-use format. Skyscape offers the best selection of PDA e-books and a great reader linking the books together. Look at their book list online and purchase the ones that will complement the recommended programs in your specialty area.

# Handheldmed and Mobipocket Reader

Handheldmed, www.handheldmed.com, is a PDA reference distributor that uses the free Mobipocket reader for all of its titles. In 2007, this company had 120 titles, including the major titles already discussed. Discounts are offered for book bundles.

## *Geriatrics at Your Fingertips*

The American Geriatric Society has developed a PDA book titled *Geriatrics at Your Fingertips (GAYF)*, and it is available in Palm and Windows versions at www.geriatricsatyourfingertips.org/front-back/pda.asp.

You must fill out an online registration and choose your version to download. A registration number will be e-mailed to you to use to unlock the program on the PDA. This is a topical problem-oriented book recommended for all students and providers who have geriatric patients. Several common problems are reviewed with guidelines, treatment tables, and assessment tools. There is a Web version that can be accessed with a Web-enabled PDA or PC at www.geriatricsatyour fingertips.org/front-back/toc.asp.

The following screen shots will demonstrate how you would use *GAYF* to help manage a geriatric patient. A video demonstration of *GAYF*, labeled Video 6–7, is available on the CD-ROM.

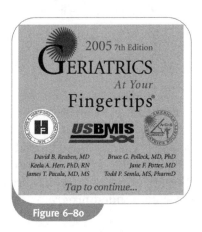

Figure 6–80

This is the opening page for *GAYF.*

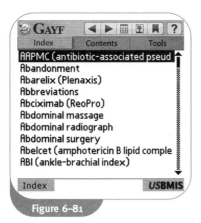

Figure 6–81

The icons across the top of the screen are:

Forward and backward buttons

Table: a list of tables

Picture: a list of figures

Bookmark: to bookmark sections

Question mark: for the program help section

The tabs show Index, Contents, and Tools. This screen is the index list of available topics.

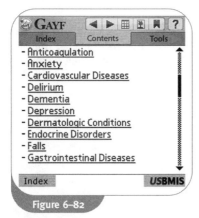

Figure 6–82

The main table of contents:

Contents: a chapter/topic listing; each topic will have an outline that users can use to navigate

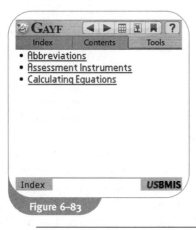

Figure 6–83

Tools is divided into three sections:

Abbreviations: used in charting

Assessment Instruments: commonly used in geriatrics

Calculating Equations: several medical calculations common to medical practice

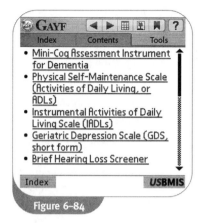

Figure 6–84

This screen displays a portion of the available Assessment Instruments. These are very helpful doing geriatric assessments in the clinic, hospital, or long-term care facility. It is great for those in internal medicine, geriatrics, or family practice.

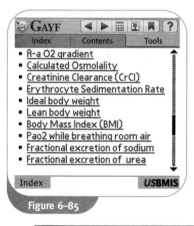

Figure 6–85

These are a few of the medical calculations available. They are helpful for any adult patient.

This PDA e-book is highly recommended by the author for students and clinicians with geriatric patients. It is very well organized and full of helpful resources.

## STAT!Ref PIER

STAT!Ref PIER on PDA is a primary care evidence-based reference product of the American College of Physicians (ACP) and is available for individual subscriptions at www.statref.com/products/PIERonPDA.html. This reference is internal medicine–primary care oriented.

The following screen shots will demonstrate how you would use STAT!Ref PIER to help manage a patient with acute low back pain. A video demonstration of Stat!Ref PIER, labeled Video 6–8, is available on the CD-ROM.

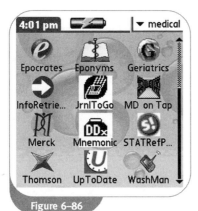

Figure 6–86

STAT!Ref PIER with the S! in the circle is the icon for this program. Tap it to start.

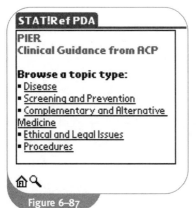

Figure 6–87

Click on the magnifying glass at the bottom of the screen to search for a topic. Or, you may choose to browse by Disease, Screening and Prevention, Complementary and Alternative Medicine, Ethical and Legal Issues, or by Procedures. These sections are unique and are not offered in other e-text-books.

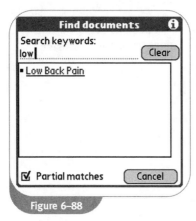

Figure 6–88

Enter the word "low" in the Search line and Low Back Pain appears in the search box results. Tap it to see the full text.

STAT!Ref PDA
Low Back Pain
Prevention
Screening
Diagnosis
Consultation for Diagnosis
Hospitalization
Non-drug Therapy
Drug Therapy
Patient Education
Consultation for Management
Follow-up
Case Scenario
Low Back Pain

Figure 6–89

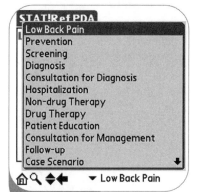

These are the topic subheadings that allow quick navigation.

---

STAT!Ref PDA
Differential Diagnosis of Low
Disease
Characteristics
Degenerative joint disease
Common radiolc abnormality th may or may no be related to symptoms
Degenerative disk disease with herniation
Common cause nerve root impingement ar
Consultation for Dic

Figure 6–90

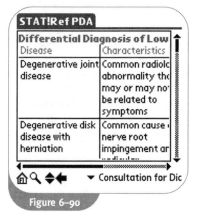

The differential diagnosis is presented as a table for review.

---

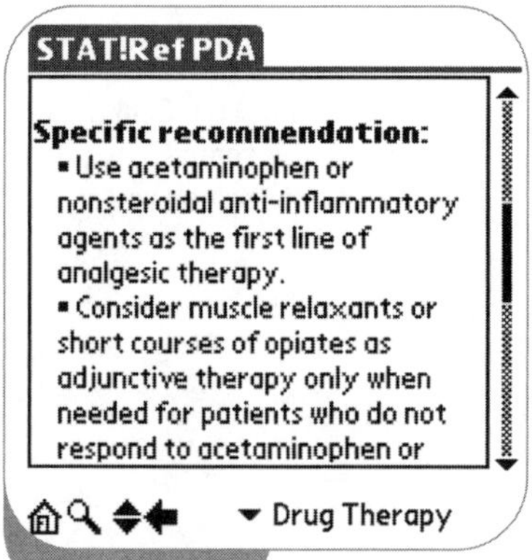

STAT!Ref PDA
Specific recommendation:
▪ Use acetaminophen or nonsteroidal anti-inflammatory agents as the first line of analgesic therapy.
▪ Consider muscle relaxants or short courses of opiates as adjunctive therapy only when needed for patients who do not respond to acetaminophen or
Drug Therapy

Figure 6–91

The treatment recommendations are given as general medication classes without drug details.

---

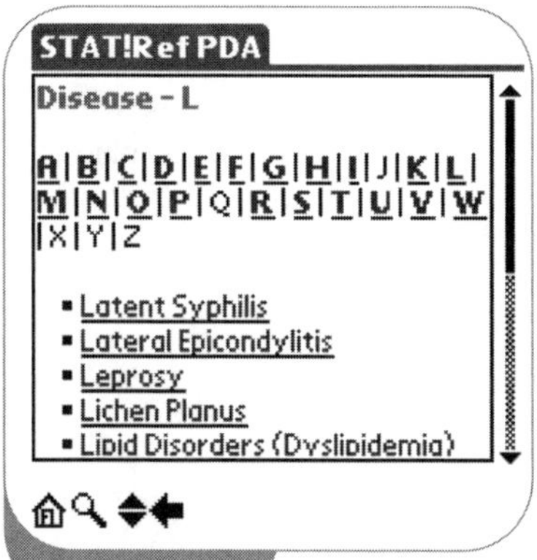

**STAT!Ref PDA**

Disease - L

A B C D E F G H I J K L
M N O P Q R S T U V W
X Y Z

- Latent Syphilis
- Lateral Epicondylitis
- Leprosy
- Lichen Planus
- Lipid Disorders (Dyslipidemia)

Figure 6-92

Do a search by disease by choosing the first letter and scrolling down the menu.

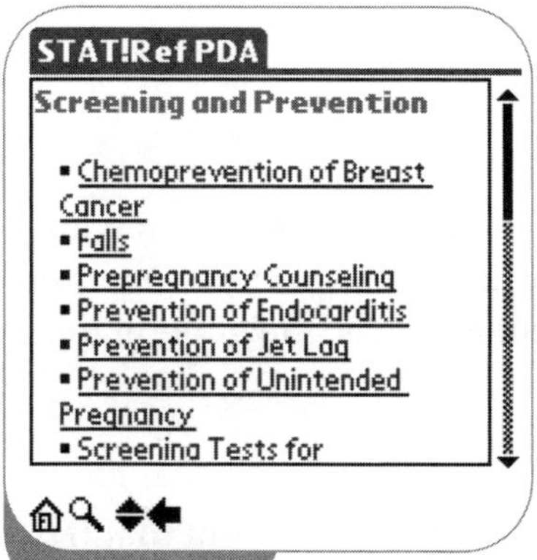

---

**STAT!Ref PDA**

**Screening and Prevention**

- Chemoprevention of Breast Cancer
- Falls
- Prepregnancy Counseling
- Prevention of Endocarditis
- Prevention of Jet Lag
- Prevention of Unintended Pregnancy
- Screening Tests for

Figure 6-93

Screening and Prevention guides are a unique feature of PIER. There are several recommendations one would encounter in an internal medicine or family practice setting.

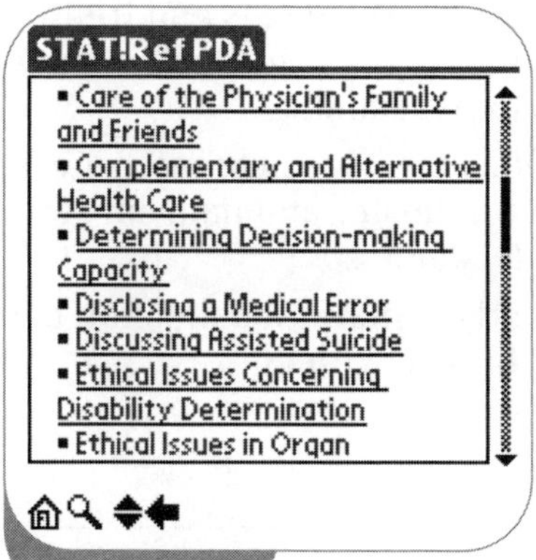

---

**STAT!Ref PDA**

- Care of the Physician's Family and Friends
- Complementary and Alternative Health Care
- Determining Decision-making Capacity
- Disclosing a Medical Error
- Discussing Assisted Suicide
- Ethical Issues Concerning Disability Determination
- Ethical Issues in Organ

Figure 6-94

The Ethical and Legal issues section also is unique. These are nice reading materials for review and quick lookups for situations that arise in practice.

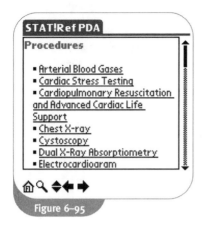

Procedures is a section with description, indications, contraindications, normal values, alert values, contraindications, and references.

Figure 6–95

STAT!Ref PIER is worth looking at if you work in internal medicine. However, check out DynaMed as well; it is the author's opinion that it might be a better buy for information on the same general topics.

## iSilo

iSilo is a PDA text reader available at http://isilo.com that has many medical and nonmedical e-book titles:

■ The Clinical Medicine Series at http://cgwebermd.tripod. com/— Quick and extensive references for the diagnosis and treatment of the majority of problems that may present in a primary care practice in iSilo or Mobipocket (free) reader.

■ MeisterMed at www.meistermed.com/—Medical references for the clinician include the free DermMeister and paid subscriptions for LyteMeister and CodeMeister.

■ The Medical iSilo Depot—Currently contains a collection of over 100 medical documents created for use with iSilo.

## Summary

Table 6-1 provides a summary of the products discussed previously in this chapter.

**Table 6-1** PDA Textbook Medical References

| Name & Web Site | Publisher/Reader | Contents | Ease/Content | 2–3 Minute Readability |
|---|---|---|---|---|
| UpToDate www.UpToDate.com | UpToDate | Own Authors | Thick content but very complete; need separate 2-GB memory card | No—you need 15 minutes at least, but great content |
| BMJ Clinical Evidence www.ClinicalEvidence.com | BMJ—Unbound Medicine | *British Medical Journal* | Informative and quick if topic present | Yes |
| Inforetriever www.InfoPOEMs.com | Wiley | 5mcc, Guidelines | Very thick and slow; information overload | No, you need 20 minutes |
| *Mobile Merck/Medicus* www.MerckMedicus.com | Unbound Medicine | *Harrison's Practice*, Diagnostic test, *Merck Manual* | Quick and informative | Yes, a must-have |
| Medicine Central www.UnboundMedicine.com | Unbound Medicine | 5mcc, Harrison's, Current Therapy | Some linking | Yes, but try free products first |
| Clinical Xpert www.ThomsonClinical Xpert.com | Thomson, PDR, and Micromedex | | Fast and helpful content | Yes, a must-have |
| Dynamed www.EBSCOhost.com/ DynaMed | SkyScape, EBSCO | Topical, like 5mcc | Quick, well-referenced write-up | Yes |

*continues*

**Table 6-1** PDA Textbook Medical References (continues)

| Name & Web Site | Publisher/Reader | Contents | Ease/Content | 2–3 Minute Readability |
|---|---|---|---|---|
| Clinical Constellation www.SkyScape.com | SkyScape | 5mcc, drug, | Slow and disjointed | No |
| Geriatrics—GAYF www.GeriatricsAtYour Fingertips.org | American Geriatric Society | Topical | Fast and informative | Yes, geriatrics |
| STAT!Ref PIER www.STATRef.com | ACP American College of Physicians | Topical reference | Fast and informative | Yes, IM based |

The textbooks available for PDA each stand on their own merits. Consider buying the PDA version instead of the paper version because of continuous updates and portability. Buy from a company that has the most titles you want so that the reader will be the same and the books will be cross linked. If possible, download a trial version and apply it in your practice before you buy.

# Teaching and Learning PDA-EBM Skills

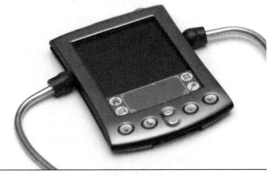

## Objectives

- Discuss the tools needed to perform classroom demonstrations.
- Practice exercises to integrate PDA use in medical curricula.
- Integrate EBM as a method of lifelong learning.

## Tools to Assist in Teaching

EBM is a strategy to promote lifelong learning, continuing medical education, and a high quality of medical care based on the latest evidence. A side benefit is continuous study review for board examinations and potential CME credits. Using PDAs to facilitate EBM practice is new to many practicing clinicians, faculty, and students. You may be the PDA leader in your practice, hospital, or school, and you may be the one called upon to lead the way and teach others. There are some software tools that will help you make presentations or educational documents.

To teach others about using their PDAs, those learning must crowd around a tiny PDA screen. A better solution, however, is to project the screen image using a standard PC projector. Some software tools make the teaching process easy.

■ PdaReach

PdaReach (www.junefabrics.com/pdareach/index.php) by June Fabrics Technology Group is a software program that runs on a PDA and laptop PC linked with the synch cable. There are Palm and Windows versions available for order. It allows you to see the PDA screen on your PC screen, enter information with your keyboard, and use the PC mouse to navigate the PDA. This program allows you to project your PC screen to a big screen by using an LCD projector connected to your PC. It comes with enlarge mode and a full-screen theater mode that is ideal for projecting the Palm screen. You can use one of several PDA skins, or pictures of various PDA screens, to look like the specific PDA device you are using.

Another useful feature from PdaReach is the support for taking screen shots, with or without any Palm skins. You easily can save any Palm screen to an image file on disk. These images are stored as bit-mapped or .bmp files that can be placed into Microsoft PowerPoint or Word documents. Palm actually uses this feature to build their training materials. The cost for an individual download as of 2008 is $24.

The following screen shots will demonstrate how you would use PdaReach to demonstrate PDA programs on a computer or big screen, or to make pictures.

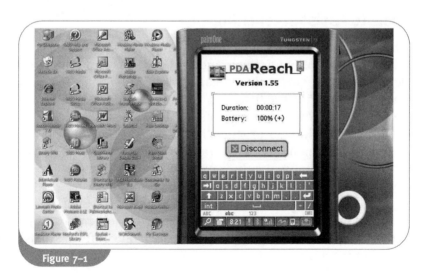

Figure 7–1

PdaReach running on a laptop computer screen.

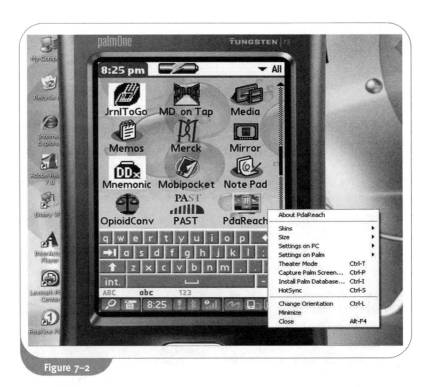

Figure 7–2

Right click over the PDA image in the middle of the screen and a menu box will appear. The options include:

Skins—Shows the different models of PDA to be displayed around the screen.

Size—Puts a single or double size picture of the PDA on the PC screen. Double size is recommended.

Settings on PC—Displays a list of options and preferences you can customize on your PC.

Settings on Palm—Displays a list of options and preferences with which you can customize on your PDA.

Install Palm Database—This allows you to install Palm Data files located on your PC. It is recommended that you install the applications you want to demonstrate directly to your PDA using the instructions provided.

HotSync—This activates the HotSync program to transfer information from your PDA to your PC.

The Theater Mode and Capture Palm Screen options are described in Figures 7–3 and 7–4.

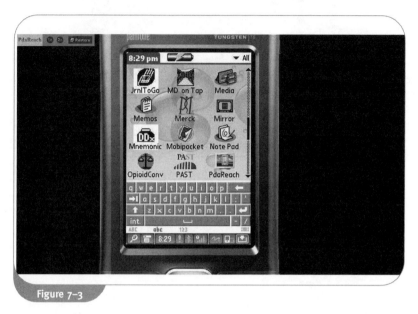

Theater Mode puts a black background behind the PDA image for optimal projection to a big screen with a PC projector.

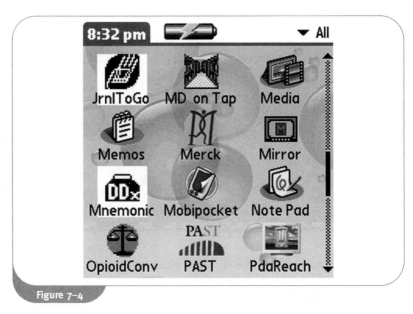

Figure 7-4

The Capture Palm Screen menu option will create a bit-mapped (.bmp) picture file of the PDA screen to use in training documents or PowerPoint slide shows. Only what you see on the PDA screen is captured; the skin is not.

■ Camtasia Studio

TechSmith's Camtasia Studio at www.techsmith.com/camtasia.asp is a screen-capture program that allows the user to make demonstration videos for distribution on CD-ROM, DVD, or streaming video from a Web site. To place a video for viewing on the Web, you would need to upload the video file to a Web video server and place the link location on a Web page. YouTube, www.youtube.com, is a popular video server available for free. Some universities have video servers for faculty and student use.

Camtasia allows the user to add audio narration to the video using a microphone plugged into the PC. Using Camtasia to create the screen capture and PdaReach to bring the PDA screen onto the PC is a great combination to produce teaching videos. There are excellent online video tutorials about using Camtasia made with the same software at www.techsmith.com/learn/default.asp.

The following screen shots demonstrate how to use Camtasia for recording PDA screens for video demonstrations.

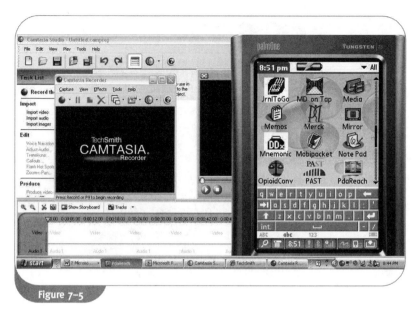

Figure 7-5

The program allows you to record all the activity in one part of the PC screen or the entire screen. This figure shows Camtasia in the background and the PDA screen obtained by using PdaReach. Camtasia allows you to draw a box around the area of the screen you want to capture, like the PDA screen, and all the activity on the PDA screen will be captured to a video file. The captured video file can be edited, narrated, put into slide shows, or placed online to be streamed from an Internet site. A video of how Camtasia works is included on the enclosed CD-ROM labeled Video 7-1.

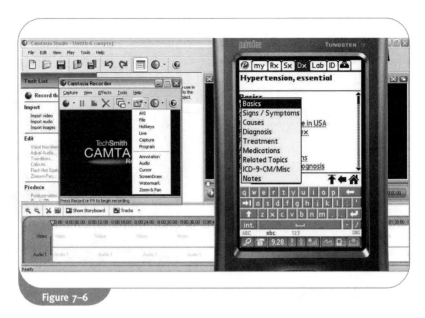

Figure 7-6

Open the Options menu by clicking on the icon of the hand in the Camtasia Recorder and click on Capture. This will open a box of capture options.

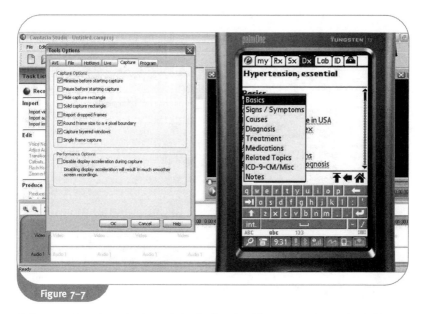

Figure 7–7

Make sure there is a check mark in the box beside Capture layered windows. This allows capture of the PDA screen video as a layered window (several open programs on one screen) on your computer screen. Now you are ready to make movies of the screen shots as you demonstrate the software. You can add audio narration after you have recorded the video. A video demonstration labeled Video 7–1 is provided on the accompanying CD-ROM.

# Using Patient Cases to Teach and Learn: "Have a Disease" Workshops

At the Emory Physician Assistant program, students learn how to do the entire medical history and physical exam in the first semester. The challenge in most medical training programs is providing practice patient encounters to help students learn medical history and physical examination skills. There are logistical problems with sending students to multiple clinical sites with mentors and there is also a cost to providing actor-patients. The purpose of adding "Have a Disease" workshops to the medical interviewing course is to give students practice doing multiple simulated patient interviews in the classroom environment. It requires no special equipment, facilities, or travel arrangements to clinical sites. In these workshops, students also learn how to use PDA resources available at the bedside. Students learn the pathophysiology, presentation signs, and symptoms, and they work up a common patient presentation. Students then provide feedback to each other on their interviewing techniques and their diagnostic accuracy.

A class is divided into four groups. Each group is assigned a disease category with a chief complaint of chest, back, head, or abdominal pain. Each student is given the assignment to learn a disease that has a primary presentation within that category. For example, if a student was assigned to the chest pain group, she could learn about myocardial infarction, angina, pulmonary embolus, and so on. The student learns about the single disease that has been chosen, including the presenting symptoms, risk factors, and family history. Each student is told to keep the disease a secret until after the assigned partner presents the diagnostic history with a differential diagnosis.

Students are taught how to perform the medical interview with in-class lectures, mnemonics, and video examples. Each section of the interview, including the history of the present illness (HPI), past medical history (PMH), family history (FH), social history (SH), and the review of systems (ROS), is practiced in class, with students role playing scenarios in groups of two. Once all the sections of the history are mastered, four 1-hour "Have a Disease" workshops are scheduled. The format for these sessions is as follows:

- Students are assigned a partner from another group. For example, the chest pain group is paired with abdominal pain group and the back pain group with the head pain group.

- Each student is given 10 minutes to do a problem-specific medical history. Students then are given 10 minutes to use their PDA resources to write a quick summary of the history and construct a ranked differential diagnosis. Students use *Diagnosaurus* and *Differential Diagnosis Mnemonics* to help construct a differential and the Dx portion of Epocrates to read about the diseases they are contemplating. For the next 15 minutes, students present the history to each other as if they were presenting to a supervising physician. At the end of this segment, each student provides written feedback on their interviewing skills and reveals the actual diagnosis they were role playing.

- For one of the four sessions, students prepare a single-page patient write-up. This includes the patient history, a ranked differential diagnosis, and a plan that includes diagnostic tests, treatment, and patient education. Students are encouraged to use their PDA resources to do this. This is graded by the faculty and returned with comments.

■ For the next session, students are paired with another group. For example, the chest pain group goes with the head pain group and the abdominal pain group with the back pain group. Each student keeps his disease secret and role plays it four times with four different partners. This gives the students a sense of clinical pursuit of the unknown and a familiarity with common patient presentations in a fun, controlled environment.

Based on their participation write-up, students are given feedback from faculty as well as a peer evaluation. The main method of student evaluation is a timed, 10-minute graded interview with a standardized patient and relating to a specific problem. The interview is monitored by a faculty member with a checklist. The students know ahead of time that the standardized patient will have one of the four chief complaints used in the workshop: chest pain, head pain, abdominal pain, or back pain. An impressive 98 percent of the first class made above 90 percent on the final. Student feedback on the workshops was positive, revealing that it was a fun and challenging way to learn and practice history skills at the same time. Through this teaching method, students learned the power of the PDA tools in an environment in which faculty could help.

## Sample Cases

These cases are common presentations that could be made to any emergency department. They are teaching examples for you to show the benefits of using PDAs with EBM software. These cases will be demonstrated in a series of videos available on the CD-ROM.

## ■ Headache

A 32-year-old female elementary school teacher presents to the emergency department with a 1-day history of frontal headache, located above both eyes and without any radiation. It is ranked a 4 on a scale of 10 in intensity. The headache is constant and feels like a pressure. The headache began at home after a week of nasal congestion. Now she has green nasal drainage. She has no history of rash, fever, chills, head injury, visual disturbances, ear ache, cough, nausea, or vomiting.

■ What is the differential diagnosis?
■ What is the best cost-effective workup?
■ What is the ICD-9 code for the top diagnosis?
■ What would the best treatment be?

A video demonstration of this case solution using Epocrates Essentials, labeled Video 7–2, is available on the CD-ROM.

## ■ Chest Pain

A 40-year-old male accountant presents to the emergency department with 2 days of increasing substernal nonradiating chest pain rated 5 on a scale of 10. The pain began after a viral syndrome that lasted for 5 days. He has had a mild fever to 101, and it hurts worse when he lays flat or takes a deep breath. There is no history of heart disease, dyspnea, PND, nausea, or vomiting.

■ What is the differential diagnosis?
■ What is the best cost-effective workup?
■ What is the ICD-9 code for the top diagnosis?
■ What would the best treatment be?

A video demonstration of this case solution using Epocrates Essentials, labeled Video 7–3, is available on the CD-ROM.

## ■ Abdominal Pain

A 40-year-old female cook presents with 2 days of colicky right upper quadrant abdominal pain, nausea, and vomiting. She has had similar pains for 2 months after eating greasy foods.

- What is the differential diagnosis?
- What is the best cost-effective workup?
- What is the ICD-9 code for the top diagnosis?
- What would the best treatment be?

A video demonstration of this case solution using Epocrates Essentials, labeled Video 7–4, is available on the CD-ROM.

■ Back Pain

A 50-year-old engineer presents with 1 week of increasing nonradiating low back pain. He is awakened at night with this dull constant pain, but it is relieved a little with ibuprofen. He has had a 10-pound weight loss over 1 month and is not dieting.

- What is the differential diagnosis?
- What is the best cost-effective workup?
- What is the ICD-9 code for the top diagnosis?
- What would the best treatment be?

A video demonstration of this case solution using Epocrates Essentials, labeled Video 7–5, is available on the CD-ROM.

■ Dyspnea

A 50-year-old female salesperson presents to the emergency department with 2 days of dyspnea on exertion and generalized edema of the feet and hands. She also has symptoms of nocturia.

- What is the differential diagnosis?
- What is the best cost-effective workup?
- What is the ICD-9 code for the top diagnosis?
- What would the best treatment be?

A video demonstration of this case solution using Epocrates Essentials, labeled Video 7–6, is available on the CD-ROM.

■ Cough

A 27-year-old male college student presents to the clinic with 3 days of productive cough, fever, and chills. The sputum is green and he states that he has a deep pain in his right chest when he coughs. He does not smoke, use street drugs, or have any HIV risk factors.

- What is the differential diagnosis?
- What is the best cost-effective workup?
- What is the ICD-9 code for the top diagnosis?
- What would the best treatment be?

A video demonstration of this case solution using Epocrates Essentials, labeled Video 7–7, is available on the CD-ROM.

- Sore Throat

A 16-year-old female has 1 week of sore throat, fatigue, fever, and malaise. There is no earache, nasal congestion, cough, headache, or rash.

- What is the differential diagnosis?
- What is the best cost-effective workup?
- What is the ICD-9 code for the top diagnosis?
- What would the best treatment be?

A video demonstration of this case solution using Epocrates Essentials, labeled Video 7–8, is available on the CD-ROM.

## Integrating PDAs into the Medical Curricula and Training Programs

It would be advantageous to all medical facilities, including teaching facilities, to have a resident computer expert who is familiar with PDA use in the medical field. This would be the ideal person to implement an EBM-PDA curriculum, whether in the classroom or in the facility itself. If there is no interest, students or medical professionals may band together and form a work group to get software discounts and share resources.

Courses on medical informatics, covering online medical records, PDAs, and Web resources, should be prevalent in the near future. Many schools currently offer this as an online self-study module or during school orientation. Current medical students should request that these new skills be integrated into the curricula to keep them competitive in the evolving job market.

PDA and EBM tools should be standard equipment when working with standardized patients. There should be a 5-minute PDA break during the history time (pager break) to allow the student to review the differential diagnosis based on the chief complaint and the history of the present illness. There should be another PDA break after the physical examination to allow the student to form a prioritized differential diagnosis and a lab, imaging, and therapy strategy.

Use the PDA and EBM tools to follow along in the classroom during clinical medicine lectures. Most programs have a note-taking feature to capture information not already listed in the EBM resources. This can lead to lively discussions if your PDA resources are more up to date than the lecturer, but it will motivate faculty to learn the tools and update their material with the latest information.

# EBM and PDA Resources

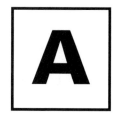

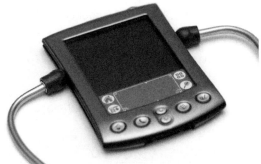

This appendix provides EBM and PDA resources and Web sites not discussed in the rest of the book.

## Evidence-Based Medicine Resources

■ EBM Web Sites

These are Web sites that have information and links to classic evidence-based medicine techniques and resources.

The Centre for Evidence-Based Medicine: http://www.cebm.net/

SUNY Downstate EBM Tutorial: http://library.downstate.edu/
   resources/ebm.htm

Michigan State University Introduction to Evidence-Based Medicine
   Course: www.poems.msu.edu/InfoMastery/

Duke University Introduction to Evidence-Based Medicine:
   www. hsl.unc.edu/services/tutorials/ebm/welcome.htm

Users' Guides to Evidence-Based Practice (Originally published as a
   series in the *Journal of the American Medical Association*):
   www. cche.net/usersguides/main.asp

Glossary of EBM Terms: http://www.ebem.org/definitions.html

Evidence-Based Emergency Medicine: www.ebem.org/index.php

Evidence-Based Medicine Toolkit: http://www.ebm.med.ualberta.ca/

■ Definitions of Levels of Evidence, Web reference

Medical reviewers making evidence-based recommendations will grade the strength of the evidence, or study results, using a uniform grading scale. Many of the Web sites and programs discussed in this book use this uniform evidence grading scale where 1 is the best and 5 is the worst. www.cebm.net/levels_of_evidence.asp

# Key to Interpretation of Practice Guidelines

■ Agency for Healthcare Research and Quality

The Agency for Healthcare Research and Quality (AHRQ) put in place twelve Evidence-based Practice Centers (EPCs) in 1997 to help integrate evidence-based medicine in frontline medical care offices. They have several EBM guidelines online at their Web site (www.ahrq.gov/clinic/epcindex.htm).

■ United States Preventive Services Task Force (USPSTF) Guide to Clinical Preventive Services

The U.S. Preventive Services Task Force (USPSTF) is made up of expert panels that produce preventive guidelines for primary care providers. The Web site is www.ahrq.gov/clinic/uspstfix.htm. They have a free PDF file for PDA download or Web book accessible with a Web-connected PDA. The Guide to Clinical Preventive Services is a pocket guide from the USPSTF with the latest recommendations for disease prevention, screening, and counseling for primary care providers.

■ Other Guidelines

Other guidelines, such as those at the National Guideline Clearing-house (www.guideline.gov), have a uniform grading scale to help the reader appraise the recommendations.

## Web Sites That May Help

This section lists several Web sites that may help provide additional information about PDA equipment, software, and tips on how to use them.

■ Medical PDA Sites

Video Tutorial on using PDAs: www.doctorsgadgets.com/the-doctors-pda-and-smartphone-handbook/

StatCoder: www.statcoder.com/

American Medical Student Association (AMSA) PDA Information: www.amsa.org/resource/pda.cfm

Medical Eponyms: www.eponyms.net/

Medical Mnemonics: www.medicalmnemonics.com

pdaMD: www.pdamd.com/home

Johns Hopkins Antibiotic Guide: www.hopkins-abxguide.org

MedCalc Free Medical Calculator: www.med-ia.ch/medcalc/

American College of Physicians PDA Portal: www.acponline.org/pda/index.html?hp

PDA Consumer Reviews: www.consumersearch.com

Florida State University Medical PDA Software: www.med.fsu.edu/library/PDASoftware.asp

Emory University Physician Assistant Program PDA Links:
www. emorypa.org/useful_links.htm

University of Virginia Medical School PDA Resource Page:
www.healthsystem.virginia.edu/internet/library/wdc-lib/services/
computing/pda/

Yale Medical PDA Resources and Services: www.med.yale.edu/
library/technology/PDA/

UConn Health Center PDA Resources: http://library.uchc.edu/pda/

Duke University Introduction to Evidence-Based Medicine:
www.hsl.unc.edu/services/tutorials/ebm/index.htm

Collective Med PDA Center: www.collectivemed.com

## Medical Guideline PDA Sites

These are Web sites of leading authorities that have PDA versions of
the latest treatment and diagnosis guidelines, and most of these resources are free. Choose the guidelines that are helpful in your daily
practice.

■ American Academy of Family Physicians

Asthma guidelines and a preventive services PDA tool are available at
the American College of Physicians Web site at www.aafp.org/online/
en/home/membership/resources/aafp-pda-downloads/clinprev.html.

■ American College of Cardiology Foundation

The American College of Cardiology has developed the ACC Info
Guide. The software application and documents listed here are available for download from the American College of Cardiology Web site
at www.acc.org/qualityandscience/clinical/palm_download.htm.

■ Pocket guideline for the management of patients with unstable
angina and non–ST-segment elevation myocardial infarction

- Pocket guideline for coronary artery bypass graft surgery (CABG)
- Pocket guideline for evaluation and management of chronic heart failure in the adult
- Pocket guideline for implantation of cardiac pacemakers and antiarrhythmia devices
- Pocket guideline for the management of patients with atrial fibrillation
- Pocket guideline for the management of patients with chronic stable angina
- Pocket guideline for perioperative cardiovascular evaluation for noncardiac surgery

## American College of Chest Physicians

The documents listed here are available for download from the American College of Chest Physicians Web site at www.chestnet.org/education/guidelines/currentGuidelines.php.

- Evidence-based assessment of diagnostic tests for ventilator-associated pneumonia
- Managing cough as a defense mechanism and as a symptom
- Pulmonary rehabilitation: Joint ACCP/AACVPR evidence-based guidelines
- Seventh ACCP Consensus Conference on Antithrombotic Therapy (2004): Summary
- Lung Cancer Diagnosis and Management

## American College of Physicians

The following references are available for download at the American College of Physicians Web site at www.acponline.org/pda/clinical_references.htm.

- Domestic violence intervention tools
- Commonly used ICD-9 codes: 2006–2007 edition
- Gynecology alerts
- Calorie-savings food list
- Normal lab values from MKSAP 12

- Vaccine-specific information
- JNC VI (1997) hypertension management
- USPSTF preventive services guidelines
- 2001 ADA guidelines
- 2001 NCEP ATP III guidelines
- Danger signs or symptoms that suggest head and neck cancer
- Drugs used in the treatment of HIV infection
- Table of normal physiological changes during pregnancy
- Obstetric medicine curriculum
- DSM-IV criteria for major depressive episode
- Pharmacotherapies for acute major depression
- Differential diagnosis between allergic and nonallergic rhinitis

### American College of Radiology

The American College of Radiology has developed the Appropriateness Criteria Anytime, Anywhere PDA application, which is available at www.acr.org/SecondaryMainMenuCategories/ACRStore/Featured Categories/QualityandSafety/ac_pda.aspx for a fee.

### American Diabetes Association

The Clinical Practice Recommendations Standards of Care is available for viewing on a Palm or pocket PC from the American Diabetes Association Web site at www.diabetes.org/for-health-professionals-and-scientists/cpr.jsp.

### American Heart Association

The American Heart Association (AHA) has made a number of its guidelines, jointly developed with the American College of Cardiology (ACC), available in PDA-downloadable format. Guidelines may be viewed with the freely distributable APPRISOR Document Viewer for Palm OS or by the iSilo document reader for Palm OS or Pocket PC OS. The APPRISOR Document Viewer, technical support information, and the following guidelines are available for download at www.apprisor.com.

- ACC/AHA pocket guideline for coronary artery bypass graft surgery

- ACC/AHA pocket guideline for implantation of cardiac pacemakers and antiarrhythmia devices
- ACC/AHA pocket guideline for management of patients with acute myocardial infarction
- ACC/AHA pocket guideline for management of patients with chronic stable angina
- ACC/AHA pocket guideline for perioperative cardiovascular evaluation for noncardiac surgery
- ACC/AHA pocket guideline for the management of patients with unstable angina and non–ST-segment elevation myocardial infarction
- ACC/AHA pocket guidelines for the management of chronic heart failure in the adult
- ACC/AHA pocket guidelines for the management of patients with atrial fibrillation
- ACC/AHA secondary guideline for consensus panel guide to comprehensive risk reduction for patients with coronary and other atherosclerotic vascular disease

- American Medical Directors Association

The documents listed here are available for download from the American Medical Directors Association (AMDA) Web site at www.amda.com/tools/guidelines.cfm.

- PDA application: depression
- PDA application: falls and fall risk
- PDA application: pain management

- Centers for Disease Control and Prevention

- TB treatment guidelines. Available for download from www.cdc.gov/tb/pubs/PDA_TBGuidelines/default.htm.

The following guidelines and related resources (when available) can be downloaded from the AIDSinfo Web site at http://aidsinfo.nih.gov/PDATools/guidelines.aspx?MenuItem=AIDSinfoTools.

- (1) Prevention and treatment of tuberculosis among patients with infected human immunodeficiency virus: Principles of therapy and revised recommendations. (2) Notice to readers: updated guidelines for the use of rifabutin or rifampin for the treatment and prevention of tuberculosis among HIV-infected patients taking protease inhibitors or nonnucleoside reverse transcriptase inhibitors. (3) Updated guidelines for the use of rifamycins for the treatment of tuberculosis among HIV-infected patients taking protease inhibitors or nonnucleoside reverse transcriptase inhibitors

■ 2001 USPHS/IDSA guidelines for the prevention of opportunistic infections in persons infected with HIV

■ Antiretroviral postexposure prophylaxis after sexual, injection-drug use, or other nonoccupational exposure to HIV in the United States: recommendations from the U.S. Department of Health and Human Services

■ Guidelines for the use of antiretroviral agents in HIV-infected adults and adolescents

■ Guidelines for the use of antiretroviral agents in pediatric HIV infection

■ Public Health Service Task Force Recommendations for the Use of Antiretroviral Drugs in Pregnant HIV-1 Infected Women for Maternal Health and Interventions to Reduce Perinatal HIV-1 Transmission in the United States

■ Updated U.S. Public Health Service guidelines for the management of occupational exposures to HIV and recommendations for postexposure prophylaxis


■ European Society of Cardiology

The pocket guidelines listed here are available for download from the European Society of Cardiology Web site at http://pocketgram.net/escardio/.

■ Acute coronary syndromes in patients presenting without ST-segment elevation

■ Acute heart failure

■ Acute myocardial infarction

■ Antiplatelet agents

■ Cardiovascular disease prevention

■ Chronic heart failure

■ Diagnosis and management of pericardial diseases

- Interpretation of the neonatal electrocardiogram
- Management of cardiovascular diseases during pregnancy
- Management of adult congenital heart disease
- Management of syncope
- Percutaneous coronary interventions
- Prevention, diagnosis, and treatment of infective endocarditis
- Prevention of sudden cardiac death
- Pulmonary arterial hypertension
- Stable angina pectoris

- National Health Care for the Homeless Council, Inc.

An outline of main points contained in the guideline "Adapting Your Practice: General Recommendations for the Care of Homeless Patients" is available for download as a PDF file from the National Health Care for the Homeless Council Web site at www.nhchc.org/Clinicians/genreccabrev.pdf.

- National Heart, Lung and Blood Institute

Asthma Treatment Guidelines for the Palm OS. U.S. Department of Health and Human Services, Public Health Service, National Institutes of Health, National Heart, Lung and Blood Institute. Available from the National Heart, Lung and Blood Institute (NHLBI) Web site at http:// hp2010.nhlbihin.net/as_palm.htm.

ATP III cholesterol management implementation tool for Palm OS. Available from the NHLBI Web site at http://hp2010.nhlbihin.net/atpiii/atp3palm.htm.

- U.S. Public Health Service

This is preventative information for clinicians.

- Quit smoking: consumer interactive tool (PDA/Palm). Rockville (MD): Agency for Healthcare Research and Quality (AHRQ); 2004. Available from the Agency for Healthcare Research and Quality (AHRQ) Web site at http://pda.ahrq.gov/consumer/qscit/qscit.htm.

■ U.S. Preventive Services Task Force

The Electronic Preventive Services Selector (ePSS), at http://epss. ahrq.gov/PDA/index.jsp and available as a PDA application and a Web-based tool, is a quick hands-on tool designed to help primary care clinicians identify the screening, counseling, and preventive medication services that are appropriate for their patients. It is based on current recommendations of the U.S. Preventive Services Task Force (USP-STF) and can be searched by specific patient characteristics, such as age, sex, and selected behavioral risk factors.

All USPSTF guidelines that are published in the *Annals of Internal Medicine* as part of the third edition of the *Guide to Clinical Preventive Services* also are available for PDA download from the *Annals of Internal Medicine* Web site at www.acponline.org/annalspdaservices/collections/index.html.

■ Aspirin for the primary prevention of cardiovascular events: recommendations and rationale

■ Behavioral counseling in primary care to promote physical activity: recommendation and rationale

■ Chemoprevention of breast cancer: recommendations and rationale

■ Genetic risk assessment and BRCA mutation testing for breast and ovarian cancer susceptibility: recommendation statement

■ Hormone therapy for the prevention of chronic conditions in postmenopausal women: recommendation statement

■ Lung cancer screening: recommendation statement

■ Routine aspirin and nonsteroidal anti-inflammatory drug (NSAID) prophylaxis for colorectal cancer prevention

■ Routine vitamin supplementation to prevent cancer and cardiovascular disease: recommendations and rationale

■ Screening and behavioral counseling interventions in primary care to reduce alcohol misuse: recommendation statement

■ Screening for abdominal aortic aneurysms: recommendation statement

■ Screening for breast cancer: recommendations and rationale

■ Screening for colorectal cancer: recommendations and rationale

■ Screening for coronary heart disease: recommendation statement

- Screening for dementia: recommendations and rationale
- Screening for depression: recommendations and rationale
- Screening for family and intimate partner violence: recommendation statement
- Screening for hemochromatosis: recommendation statement
- Screening for hepatitis C in adults: recommendation statement
- Screening for HIV: recommendation statement
- Screening for obesity in adults: recommendations and rationale
- Screening for prostate cancer: recommendations and rationale
- Screening for suicide risk: recommendation statement
- Screening for thyroid disease: recommendation statement
- Screening for type 2 diabetes mellitus in adults: recommendations and rationale

- General PDA Web Resources

Glossary of PDA Terms: www.handango.com/Glossary.jsp

PDA Consumer Reviews: www.brighthand.com/reviews/

CNET.com PDAs: www.cnet.com/4244-5_1-0.html?query=PDA&tag=srch&target=nw

ZDNet PDA Reviews: http://review.zdnet.com/Reviews/4566-3127_16-0.html

## Additional Resources

- Medical Books About PDAs

The books listed here are additional resources for medical applications using PDAs. There are some general "how to use" PDA books available, but the tutorials that come with the PDA and online resources will usually meet the needs of most users.

Al-Ubaydli, Mohammad. 2006. *The Doctor's PDA and Smartphone Handbook,* 1st edition. London, UK: Royal Society of Medicine Press.

Al-Ubaydli, Mohammad. 2003. *Handheld Computers for Doctors.* London: John Wiley & Sons.

Helopoulos, Chris. 2004. *The Medical Professional's Guide to Handheld Computing.* Sudbury, MA: Jones and Bartlett Publishers, Inc.

Strayer, Scott, Reynolds, Peter, and Ebell, Mark. 2005. *Handhelds in Medicine: A Practical Guide for Clinicians.* New York: Springer Publishing Co.

# Print Resources for PDAs

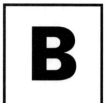

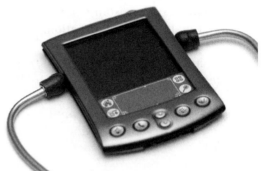

This listing is a resource for medical educators and administrators about the use of PDAs when teaching clinicians about evidence-based medicine. There are several studies demonstrating the effectiveness of PDAs.

Adatia F, Bedard PL. Palm reading: 2. Handheld software for physicians. *Can Med Assoc J.* 2003;168:727–34.

Adatia FA, Bedard PL. Palm reading: 1. Handheld hardware and operating systems. *Can Med Assoc J.* 2002;167:775–80.

Barrett JR, Strayer SM, Schubart JR. Assessing medical residents' usage and perceived needs for personal digital assistants. *Int J Med Inf.* 2004;73:25–34.

Barrett JR, Strayer SM, Schubart JR. Information needs of residents during inpatient and outpatient rotations: identifying effective personal digital assistant applications. *Proc AMIA Symp.* 2003;784. Abstract available at: www.amia.org/pubs/proceedings/symposia/start.html.

Barton, H. DynaMed. *Journal of the Medical Library Association.* 2005 Jul;93(3):412–4.

Bass SG. Wireless computing. Medical students and mobile medicine. *MD Comput.* 2000;17:27.

Beasley BW. Utility of palmtop computers in a residency program: a pilot study. *South Med J.* 2002;95:207–11.

Bertling CJ, Simpson DE, Hayes AM, Torre D, Brown DL, Schubot DB. Personal digital assistants herald new approaches to teaching and evaluation in medical education. *WMJ.* 2003;102:46–50.

Bodenheimer T, Grumbach K. Electronic technology: a spark to revitalize primary care? *JAMA.* 2003 Jul 9; 290(2):259–64.

Bower DJ, Bertling CJ. Using PalmPilots as a teaching tool during a primary care clerkship. Advanced Education Group. *Acad Med.* 2000; 75:541–2.

Briggs B. Pushing data out to PDAs. *Health Data Manag.* 2002;10:28–30.

Brilla R, Wartenberg KE. Introducing new technology: handheld computers and drug databases. A comparison between two residency programs. *J Med Syst.* 2004;28:57–61.

Brooks WB, Zbehlik A, Lurie J, Ross JM. Getting evidence based medicine to the bedside—from journal club to handheld computer. *J Gen Intern Med.* 2002;17(suppl 1):84.

Calabretta N, Fitzpatrick RB. DynaMed at the point of care. *Journal of Electronic Resources in Medical Libraries.* 2005; 2(1):55–64.

Carroll AE, Christakis DA. Pediatricians' use of and attitudes about personal digital assistants. *Pediatrics.* 2004;113:238–42.

Chen ES, Mendonca EA, McKnight LK, Stetson PD, Lei J, Cimino JJ. PalmCIS: a wireless handheld application for satisfying clinician information needs. *J Am Med Inform Assoc.* 2004;11:19–28.

Chesanow N. Colleagues rate the leading software. *Med Econ.* 2000; 77:105–8.

Clauson KA, Seamon MJ, Clauson AS, Van TB. Evaluation of drug information databases for personal digital assistants. *Am J Health Syst Pharm.* 2004 May 15;61(10):1015–24.

Criswell DF, Parchman ML. Handheld computer use in U.S. family practice residency programs. *J Am Med Inform Assoc.* 2002;9:80–6.

Dong P, Mondry A. Enhanced quality and quantity of retrieval of critically appraised topics using the CAT Crawler. *Med Inform Internet Med.* 2004 Mar;29(1):43–55.

Ebell MH. Point-of-care information that changes practice: it's closer than we think. *Family Medicine.* 2003 Apr;35(4):261–3.

Fischer S, Stewart TE, Mehta S, Wax R, Lapinsky SE. Handheld computing in medicine. *J Am Med Inform Assoc.* 2003;10:139–49.

Garvin R, Otto F, McRae MA. Using handheld computers to document family practice resident procedure experience. *Fam Med.* 2000;32: 115–8.

Gillingham W, Holt A, Gillies J. Hand-held computers in healthcare: what software programs are available? *NZ Med J.* 2002;U115:U185.

Grad RM, Meng Y, Bartlett G, Dawes M, Pluye P, Boillat M, Rao G, Thomas R. Effect of a PDA-assisted evidence-based medicine course on knowledge of common clinical problems. *Fam Med.* 2005 Nov–Dec;37(10): 734–40.

Greenberg R. Use of the personal digital assistant (PDA) in medical education. *Med Educ.* 2004;38:570–1.

Helwig AL, Flynn C. Using palm-top computers to improve students' evidence-based decision making. *Acad Med.* 1998;73:603–4.

Ho WL, Forman J, Kannry J. Portable digital assistant use in a medicine teaching program. *Proc AMIA Symp.* 2000;1031. Abstract available at: www.amia.org/pubs/proceedings/symposia/start.html.

Johnston JM, Leung GM, Tin KY, Ho LM, Lam W, Fielding R. Evaluation of a handheld clinical decision support tool for evidence-based learning and practice in medical undergraduates. *Med Educ.* 2004 Jun;38(6):628–37.

Joy S, Benrubi G. Personal digital assistant use in Florida obstetrics and gynecology residency programs. *South Med J.* 2004;97:430–3.

Kho A, Kripalani S, Dressler D, et al. Personal digital assistants at the point of care: a training program for medical students. *J Gen Intern Med.* 2004;19(suppl 1):92.

Labkoff SE, Shah S, Bormel J, Lee Y, Greenes RA. The Constellation Project: experience and evaluation of personal digital assistants in the clinical environment. *Proc Ann Symp Computer Appl Med Care.* 1995:678–82.

Lenga I, Straus S. Evidence based medicine at the point of care. *J Gen Intern Med.* 2002;17(suppl 1):201.

Leung GM, Johnston JM, Tin KY, et al. Randomised controlled trial of clinical decision support tools to improve learning of evidence based medicine in medical students. *BMJ.* 2003;327:1090–5.

Kurth RJ, Silenzio V, Irigoyen MM. Use of personal digital assistants to enhance educational evaluation in a primary care clerkship. *Med Teach.* 2002;24:488–90.

Manning B, Gadd CS. Introducing handheld computing into a residency program: preliminary results from qualitative and quantitative inquiry. *Proc AMIA Symp.* 2001;428–32.

McAlearney AS, Schweikhart SB, Medow MA. Doctors' experience with handheld computers in clinical practice: qualitative study. *BMJ.* 2004;328:1162.

McCord G, Smucker WD, Selius BA, Hannan S, Davidson E, Schrop SL, Rao V, Albrecht P. Answering questions at the point of care: do residents practice EBM or manage information sources? *Acad Med.* 2007 Mar;82(3):298–303.

McKenney RR. The next level of distributed learning: the introduction of the personal digital assistant. *J Oncol Manag.* 2004;13:18–25.

McLeod TG, Ebbert JO, Lymp JF. Survey assessment of personal digital assistant use among trainees and attending physicians. *J Am Med Inform Assoc.* 2003;10:605–7.

Mitchell JL, Sebastian J, Simpson DE. Providing students feedback: opportunity knocks in the ambulatory setting. *J Gen Intern Med.* 2002; 17(suppl 1):231.

Moffett SE, Menon AS, Meites EM, et al. Preparing doctors for bedside computing. *Lancet.* 2003;362:86.

Moore L, Richardson BR, Williams RW. The USU medical PDA initiative: the PDA as an educational tool. *Proc AMIA Symp.* 2002;528–32.

Nyun M, Aronovitz JR, Khare R, Finkelstein J. Feasibility of a palmtop based interactive education to promote safety. *Proc AMIA Symp.* 2003;955. Abstract available at: www.amia.org/pubs/proceedings/symposia/start.html.

Rao G. Introduction of handheld computing to a family practice residency program. *J Am Board Fam Pract.* 2002;15:118–22.

Rothschild JM, Lee TH, Bae T, Bates DW. Clinician use of a palmtop drug reference guide. *J Am Med Inform Assoc.* 2002;9:223–9.

Sackett, DL, Richardson, WS, Rosenberg, W, and Haynes, RB, Ed. 1997. *Evidence-Based Medicine: How to Practice and Teach EBM,* 1st ed. New York: Churchill-Livingstone, p. 2.

Schamp, RO. Your clinical questions answered. *Family Practice Management.* 2005 Nov–Dec;12(10):23.

Schwartz K, Northrup J, Israel N, Crowell K, Lauder N, Neale AV. Use of on-line evidence-based resources at the point of care. *Family Medicine.* 2003 Apr; 35(4):251–6.

Slawson D, Shaughnessy AF. Teaching evidence-based medicine: Should we be teaching information management instead? *Academic Medicine.* 2005 Jul;80(7):685–9.

Sousa AC, Zaroukian MH. Handheld computing by resident physicians: enhancing performance and demonstrating competence. *Semin Med Prac.* 2003;6:21–32.

Speedie S, Pacala J, Vercellotti G, Harris I, Zhou X. PDA support for outpatient clinical clerkships: mobile computing for medical education. *Proc AMIA Symp.* 2001;632–6. Abstract available at: www.amia.org/ pubs/proceedings/symposia/start.html.

Sullivan L, Halbach JL, Shu T. Using personal digital assistants in a family medicine clerkship. *Acad Med.* 2001;76:534–5.

Torre D, Sebastian J, Simpson DE. High impact learning activities: perceptions of third year medical students. *J Gen Intern Med.* 2003; 18(suppl 1):257.

Torre D, Sebastian J, Simpson DE, et al. Third-year medical students' perceptions of high quality learning activities across internal medicine and family medicine clerkships. *J Gen Intern Med.* 2004;18 (suppl 1): 227–8.

Torre D, Simpson DE, Sebastian J, Konicek B, Geck R, Schwantes S. Prioritizing your inpatient teaching and feedback activities. *J Gen Intern Med.* 2004;19(suppl 1):198–9.

Torre DM, Wright SM. Clinical and educational uses of handheld computers. *South Med J.* 2003;96:996–9.

Tschopp M, Lovis C, Geissbuhler A. Understanding usage patterns of handheld computers in clinical practice. *Proc AMIA Symp.* 2002; 806–9.

Van Wave TW, Dewey AK. Do medical students need a hand up on palm technology? *Minn Med.* 2003;86:18–9.

Walpert B. The operating system debate: Pocket PC vs. Palm. *ACP Observer.* 2002 Nov.

Weissman PF. A primary-care curriculum: can clinical practice guidelines be taught using active learning techniques? *J Gen Intern Med.* 2003;18(suppl 1):124.

Zaroukian MH, Sousa A. Handheld computing in resident education: benefits, barriers, and considerations. *Semin Med Prac.* 2002;5:33–44.

# Index

## A

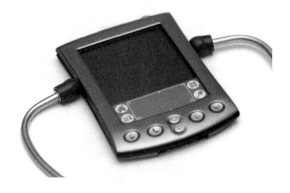

## B

InfoRetriever and InfoPOEMs, 102, *103–104*

Medicine Central, 111, *111–113*

*Mobile* Merck*Medicus* and Merck Manual, 105–106, *106–110*

STAT!Ref PIER, 132, *133–136*

UpToDate, 92–93, *93–98*

risk for disability question and, in Clinical Constellation, *129*

sample case: differential diagnosis, cost-effective workup, ICD-9 code, and best treatment in, 150

topic subheadings in *Mobile* Merck*Medicus, 107*

Bandolier, 84

home page, *84*

Search Results page, *85*

table showing likelihood ratios for headache symptoms, *85*

Bar code readers, 20

Basics page for acute low back pain, in Clinical Constellation, *125*

Battery life, PDA selection and, 20

Beaming, PDA selection and, 22

Bed rest screen, with UpToDate, *96*

Bedside, learning to use PDA resources at, 146

*Bedside Diagnosis,* 41

alphabetical list of topics in, *41*

home page, *83*

Web site, 41

BestBETs (Best Evidence Topic database), 86, *87–88*

home page, *87*

results page, *88*

search options choices, *87*

Search page, *87*

summary of recommendation and references, *88*

BestDx/BestRx, main menu, AvantGo, *70*

Best Tests section, AvantGo, *70*

Billing, future PDA scenario and, 15

Bioterrorism threats, 911 and latest information on, 122

Bluetooth, Wi-fi vs., 22–23

BMJ Clinical Evidence, 99, *100–101*

main menu page, *99*

medications list, *101*

nondrug treatment recommendations, *101*

referenced review of non-drug treatments, *101*

Topic Index, *100*

Treatment Summary, *100*

.bmp files, Palm screen images stored as, 140

Board examinations, preparing for, 14

*British Medical Journal,* 99

Business cards (electronic), beaming, 22

Business expenses, tracking, 26

## C

CABG. *See* Coronary bypass graft surgery

Calculating Equations section, *Geriatrics at Your Fingertips, 131*

Calculator function, with Clinical Xpert, *117*

Calculators, PDA, 25

Calculator symbol, in PEPID, *58*

Calendar function, logging time and title of CME functions and, 14

CAM database, Epocrates Essentials, *47*

Camtasia

in background, and PDA screen obtained by using PdaReach, *144*

Capture layered windows, *146*

capture options, *145*

using for recording PDA screens for video demonstrations, 143, *144–146*

video tutorials about, 143

Camtasia Studio, 143, *144–146*

Capture layered windows, Camtasia, *146*

Capture options, with Camtasia, *145*

Capture Palm Screen option, Pda Reach, 142, *143*

Causes and Risk Factors section, in DynaMed, 118

CC. *See* Chief complaint

CDC. *See* Centers for Disease Control and Prevention

CDC Spotlights tool, in Clinical Constellation, *124*

*Cecil Textbook of Medicine,* 106

## D

Digital cameras, secure digital (SD) memory cards and, 21
Digital pictures, 26
Disease-association tool, with PubMed, 73
Disease reference, Epocrates Essentials *vs.* PEPID, 44*t*
Disease text menu structure, in PEPID, *59*
DocAlert clinical messaging, with Epocrates Essentials, 46
Doctor's bag icon, DDx with, *31*
Doctor's bag icon, Epocrates Essentials, *47*
*Doctor's PDA and Smartphone Handbook, The* (Al-Ubaydli), 163
Documents to Go, 14, 15, 25
Dosage calculator
  in Epocrates Essential, *54, 55*
  in PEPID, *62*
Down arrow
  in DynaMed, *120*
  in PEPID, *58*
Drug and CAM therapy database, Epocrates Essentials, *47*
Drug database
  by Lexicomp, with UpToDate, *97*
  PEPID, 57–58, *62*
Drug-drug interaction feature
  caution text box in symptom analyzer, *8*
  with Epocrates Essentials, *56*
Drug information
  in Clinical Constellation, *126*
  options for, in PEPID, *61*
Drug Interaction Detail screen, in PEPID, *64*
Drug interactions
  calculating in Epocrates Essentials, *56*
  PEPID and
    calculating, *63*
    module with, 58
    in order of importance, *63*
Drug links, with Clinical Xpert, *117*
Drug multicheck program, opening, in symptom analyzer, *8*
Drug references
  with Epocrates Essentials, 46
  Epocrates Essentials *vs.* PEPID, 45*t*

with PEPID, 58
with UpToDate, by Lexicomp, *93*
Duke University, 11
Duke University Introduction to Evidence-Based Medicine, 153
  Web site for, 156
Duration selection, in symptom analyzer, *4*
DVDs, converting to video files, 27
Dx (5-Minute Clinical Consult)
  Epocrates Essentials and, *5*, 14, *47, 49*
  pulmonary embolism workup with, *50*
DXplain, 35, 36
DynaMed, 13, 118–119, *120–122*, 136, 137*t*
  disease summary sections in, 118–119
  History and Physical Examination screen, *121*
  Skyscape interface, *120*
  starting program, *120*
  submenu for acute low back pain, *121*
  Treatment section of acute low back pain menu, *122*
DynaMed caduceus, clicking on, to start program, *120*
Dyspnea sample case, differential diagnosis, cost-effective workup, ICD-9 code, and best treatment in, 150

# E

EBM. *See* Evidence-based medicine
EBM-PDAs, recommendations for, 23
EBM tools, integration of, into medical curricula and training programs, 151–152
e-books (electronic books), 3
  with chapters in eMedicine, *82*
  free trials for, 91
  saving Web references as, with AvantGo, *72*
EKG results, obtaining with Epocrates Essentials, *52*
EKG symbol, in PEPID, *58*
Electronic business cards, beaming, 22
Electronic Preventive Services Selector, 162
e-mail
  PDAs and, 25–26
  services for, 17

## F

## G



## H

Hot spots, 22
HotSync option, PdaReach, 141, *141*
House icon, in *Clinical Methods, 39*
HPI. *See* History of present illness
Hypertension
    headache and, 1–2
    sumatriptan and, *9*

# I

Ibuprofen, alternatives to, for migraine
    pain, *8*
ICD-9 codes
    in DynaMed, 118, *121*
    Epocrates Essentials *vs.* PEPID, 45*t*
    lookup reference, in Clinical Constel-
        lation, *124*
    obtaining with Epocrates Essential,
        *51*
    in PEPID, *65, 66*
Icons
    AvantGo, *69*
    CE, 99
    Clinical, in Clinical Constellation, *123*
    doctor's bag, *31, 47*
    Epocrates Essentials Main Medical
        application screen, *47*
    *Geriatrics at Your Fingertips, 131*
    InfoRetriever, *102*
    medical application, 28
    mortar, in PEPID, *58*
    question mark, in PEPID, *58*
    STAT!Ref PIER, *133*
Images, storage of, with UpToDate, *98*
Imaging approach, with UpToDate, *95,
    96*
Imaging tests, ordering with Epocrates
    Essentials, *51*
Infectious disease outbreaks, 911 and
    latest information on, 122
Infectious disease tool
    with Epocrates Essentials, 46, *47*
    Epocrates Essentials *vs.* PEPID, 45*t*
InfoPOEMs, 102
    Epocrates Essentials and, 46
InfoRetriever, 13, 14, 102, *102–104,* 137*t*
    back pain symptoms search, *103*
    Decision Support, *104*

opening screen, *102*
practice guidelines for acute low
    back pain, *104*
search options types, *103*
InfoRetriever icon, *102*
Infrared beaming ports (IrDA), 22
Install Palm Database, PdaReach, 141, *141*
Integrated EBM programs, 43–66
    Epocrates Essentials, 46–57
    PEPID, 57–66
    summary of, 66
Integrated PDA medical programs, 13
Integrated programs, description of,
    43–44
Interactive learning and testing, with
    PDA-Web connections, 15
Internet, 2, 21
    e-textbooks via, 3
    high-speed access to, 22
    latest medical evidence on, 13
Internet browsers, Web clipping and,
    67–69
Internet resources, for Web-enabled
    PDAs, 67
Interpretation screen, in Epocrates
    Essentials, *53*
Intravenous incompatibilities list, in
    Epocrates Essentials, *56*
iSilo document reader, 136, 158
IV button, in Epocrates Essentials, *56*

# J

Jaundice
    differential diagnosis of
        *Bedside Diagnosis,* 41, *41*
        *Clinical Methods,* 39, *39–40*
        *Diagnosaurus,* 33, *33–35*
        *Differential Diagnosis Mnemonics,*
            *31–32*
        Epocrates Sx, 36, *36–38*
JNC VII hypertension guidelines, in
    Tables section of symptom
    analyzer, *10*
Johns Hopkins Antibiotic Guide Web
    site, 155
Journals
    abstracts of, in *Mobile* Merck*Medicus,*
        *108*

American College of Physicians Journal Club and, 83, *83–84*

Dynamed's monitoring of, 119

reviews of, 3

watch services for, 13

j-peg (.jpg) format, 26

June Fabrics Technology Group, 140

# L

Lab menu, in Epocrates Essentials, *52*

Laboratory Resources, in Clinical Constellation, *124*

Laboratory tests, PEPID, *60*

Lab reference, Epocrates Essentials, 46, *47*

Laptop screen, PdaReach running on, *140*

Learning, with patient cases, 146–151

Licensure, CME functions on PDA and, 14

Lifelong learning, promoting, 3, 11, 14

Link button, in DynaMed, *120*

LOCATES aspects, 30

Low back pain submenu, in Clinical Constellation, *127*

LyteMeister, 136

# M

Main Medical application screen, Epocrates Essentials, *47*

Manchester Royal Infirmary (United Kingdom), BestBETs database and, 86

Massachusetts General Hospital, 35

MD on Tap, 77

for Palm or Windows, downloading, 73

PICO-formatted menu, 77

Profile section and search limits, 77

MedAlert, 123

in Clinical Constellation, *124*

MedCalc Free Medical Calculator Web site, 155

Medical application icons, 28

Medical calculators

with Epocrates Essentials, 46

Epocrates Essentials *vs.* PEPID, *45t*

with PEPID, 57–58

Medical curricula, integrating PDAs into, 151–152

Medical education, continuing, 14. *See also* Continuing medical education (CME) credits

Medical Eponyms Web site, 155

Medical evidence, acquiring latest, 13

Medical guideline PDA Web sites, 156–163

Medical history skills, "Have a Disease" workshops and, 146

Medical informatics, 151

Medical iSilo Depot, 136

Medical knowledge, exponential increase in, 11

Medical Letter, 122

Medical Mnemonics Web site, 155

Medical PDA Web sites, 155–156

*Medical Professional's Guide to Handheld Computing* (Helopoulos), 164

MedicalStudent.com, 82

Medical submenus, in PEPID, *65*

Medical textbooks, free, 80

Medical Web sites

PDA-friendly, 80–90

American College of Physicians Journal Club, 83

Bandolier, 84, *84–85*

BestBETs, 86, *87–88*

Cochrane Collection, 82–83

eMedicine, 80–82, *82*

MedicalStudent.com, 82

National Guideline Clearinghouse Web site, 88, *89–90*

Turning Research into Practice, 85, *86*

UConn Health Center Medical Library links, 82

Medication errors, reducing, 11

Medications, for migraine prevention, 7

Medications list, with BMJ Clinical Evidence, *101*

Medicine Central, 43, 111, *112–113*, 137t

*Davis's Drug Guide* link in, *113*

*Diagnosaurus* differential diagnosis for low back pain in, *112*

drug information screen in *Davis's Drug Guide* for naproxen in, *113*

## N

## Q



## R



## S

## T



## U

## V



## W



## Y



## Z

# Credits

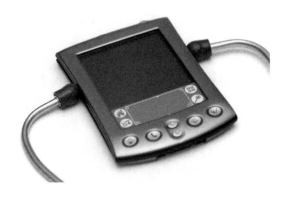

### Chapter 1

Figure 1–1 through Figure 1–20 (pp. 3–10): Courtesy of Epocrates, Inc., © 2007, All rights reserved.

### Chapter 3

Figure 3–6 through Figure 3–9 (pp. 34–35): Diagnosaurus by Roni Zieger, © 2005, The McGraw-Hill Companies, Inc.

Figure 3–10 through Figure 3–15 (pp. 36–38): Courtesy of Epocrates, Inc., © 2007, All rights reserved.

Figure 3–21 through Figure 3–22 (p. 41): Courtesy of Bedside Diagnosis, Schneiderman, Henry, 3rd edition. American College of Physicians.

### Chapter 4

Figure 4–2 through Figure 4–27 (pp. 47–57): Courtesy of Epocrates, Inc., © 2007, All rights reserved.

Figure 4–28 through Figure 4–51 (pp. 58–66): Courtesy of PEPID, LLC.

### Chapter 5

Figure 5–2 through Figure 5–8 (pp. 69–72): Courtesy of AvantGo, Sybase365.

Figure 5–27 through Figure 5–28 (pp. 81–82): Image courtesy of eMedicine.com, © 2007.

Figure 5–29 through Figure 5–30 (pp. 83–84): Bedside Diagnosis, American College of Physicians.

Figure 5–31 through Figure 5–33 (pp. 84–85): Courtesy of Bandolier.

Figure 5–34 through Figure 5–35 (p. 86): Courtesy of Trip Database.

Figure 5–36 through Figure 5–40 (p. 87–88): Courtesy of Best Bets.

**Chapter 6**

Figure 6–1 through Figure 6–16 (pp. 93–98): Reproduced with permission from UpToDate, Rose, BD (ed.). UpToDate, Waltham, MA, © 2007 UpToDate, Inc. For more information visit www.uptodate.com.

Figure 6–17 through Figure 6–22 (pp. 99–101): *BMJ Clinical Evidence*, Courtesy of BMJ Publishing Group Limited.

Figure 6–23 through Figure 6–29 (pp. 102–104): InfoRetriever-InfoPoems. Reprinted with permission of John Wiley & Sons, Inc.

Figure 6–30 through Figure 6–40 (pp. 106–110): Used with permission of Merck & Co., Inc., publishers of Merck*Medicus*. All rights reserved. Merck*Medicus* is a trademark of Merck & Co., Inc.

Figure 6–41 through Figure 6–46 (pp. 111–113): Courtesy of Unbound Medicine.

Figure 6–48 through Figure 6–57 (pp. 115–118): Reprinted with permission © 1974–2007 Thomson Healthcare. All rights reserved. The following information is an educational aid only. It is not intended as medical advice for individual conditions or treatments. Talk to your doctor, nurse or pharmacist before following any medical regimen to see if it is safe and effective for you.

Figure 6–59 through Figure 6–62 (pp. 120–122): Courtesy of DynaMed, EBSCO Publishing.

Figure 6–64 through Figure 6–79 (pp. 124–129): Clinical Constellation™ courtesy of Skyscape.

Figure 6–80 through Figure 6–85 (pp. 130–132): Courtesy of Geriatrics At Your Fingertips™, American Geriatrics Society.

Figure 6–87 through Figure 6–95 (pp. 133–136): Courtesy of STATRef, Teton Data Systems and the Physicians' Information and Education Resource (PIER), http://pier.acponline.org, Philadelphia, American College of Physicans, 2007.

## Chapter 7

Figure 7–1 through Figure 7–4 (pp. 140–143): June Fabrics PDA Technology Group, June Fabrics Technology Inc.

Figure 7–5 through Figure 7–7 (pp. 144–146): Courtesy of Tech-Smith's Camtasia Studio.